Applying

THE OCCUPATIONAL THERAPY
PRACTICE FRAMEWORK

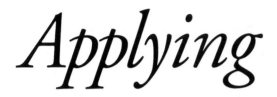

Applying
THE OCCUPATIONAL THERAPY
PRACTICE FRAMEWORK

The Cardinal Hill Occupational Participation Process

Camille Skubik-Peplaski, MS, OTR/L, BCP
Chasity Paris, MS, OTR/L
Dana Rae Collins Boyle, OTR/L
Amy Culpert, OTR/L

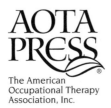

AOTA PRESS

The American
Occupational Therapy
Association, Inc.

Vision Statement

The American Occupational Therapy Association advances occupational therapy as the pre-eminent profession in promoting the health, productivity, and quality of life of individuals and society through the therapeutic application of occupation.

Mission Statement

The American Occupational Therapy Association advances the quality, availability, use, and support of occupational therapy through standard-setting, advocacy, education, and research on behalf of its members and the public.

AOTA Staff

Frederick P. Somers, Executive Director

Christopher M. Bluhm, Chief Operating Officer

Audrey Rothstein, Director, Marketing and Communications

Chris Davis, Managing Editor, AOTA Press

Barbara Dickson, Production Editor

Deborah Lieberman, MHSA, OTR/L, FAOTA, Program Director, Evidence-Based Practice

Robert A. Sacheli, Manager, Creative Services

Sarah E. Ely, Book Production Coordinator

Marge Wasson, Marketing Manager

Elizabeth Johnson, Marketing Specialist

The American Occupational Therapy Association, Inc.
4720 Montgomery Lane
Bethesda, MD 20814
Phone: 301-652-AOTA (2682)
TDD: 800-377-8555
Fax: 301-652-7711
www.aota.org
To order: 1-877-404-AOTA (2682)

Disclaimers

This publication is designed to provide accurate and authoritative information in regard to the subject matter covered. It is sold or distributed with the understanding that the publisher is not engaged in rendering legal, accounting, or other professional service. If legal advice or other expert assistance is required, the services of a competent professional person should be sought.
—*From the Declaration of Principles jointly adopted by the American Bar Association and a Committee of Publishers and Associations*

It is the objective of the American Occupational Therapy Association to be a forum for free expression and interchange of ideas. The opinions expressed by the contributors to this work are their own and not necessarily those of the American Occupational Therapy Association.

ISBN: 1-56900-216-9

Library of Congress Control Number: 2006920220

Design by Sarah E. Ely
Composition by The Electronic Quill, Silver Spring, Maryland
Printed by Versa Press, Inc., East Peoria, Illinois

Contents

Figures and Tables

Introduction

A Historical Perspective of Occupational Therapy in Rehabilitation

In the early 1900s, individuals with disabilities were isolated from society and cared for in the home by family members because of the prevailing negative attitudes regarding people with disabilities (Seidel, 1998). These family members came together and facilitated the shift of care of individuals with disabilities from the home to the community, which led to the development of rehabilitation facilities. At the same time, early occupational therapists were working as reconstruction aides who provided occupation-based activities for individuals with disabilities. Occupational therapists began working in the rehabilitation setting in the mid-1930s in response to the needs of individuals who were injured in World War I and in response to the emerging field of physical medicine. Occupational therapists prepared these injured soldiers both physically and psychologically for vocational training. Participation in war efforts gave the field of occupational therapy increased recognition and a position within the medical and military arenas (Colman, 1992). The emergence of "physical medicine was able to offer occupational therapy a certain level of clinical status it had not previously known" (p. 65).

After World War II, rehabilitation became a specialty area in which individuals in a facility were taught how to function as independently as possible in their daily living activities, instead of just providing shelter or basic care (Seidel, 1998). Occupational therapists played a crucial role in increasing independence in individuals with disabilities because "chronic illness and diseases became more prevalent and medical advances enabled people to survive accidents and traumatic injuries with permanent disabilities" (p. 537). After World War II, advances in science and new theories provided new treatment mediums for occupational therapists and more opportunities to specialize in new areas such as neurorehabilitation (Schwartz, 1998). Occupational therapists began to specialize in rehabilitation because of the increased demand for occupational therapy in response to the emergence of a community model, the deinstitutionalization of individuals with chronic illness or disability, and the large number of soldiers returning home with permanent physical injuries (Seidel, 1998). Both World War I and World War II helped "increase public awareness of the benefits of occupational therapy and provided an opportunity for therapists to prove their competence and social worth" (Schwartz, 1998, p. 857). These benefits opened the door for the profession to be a valuable service that was reimbursable by insurance and worthy of continued funding for research to improve the satisfaction and well-being of all individuals receiving occupational therapy intervention.

With these advantages came turmoil as the doctors of physical medicine (physiatrists) strived to control the education and training of occupational therapists. The problem was that the physiatrists followed the medical model, in which the focus was on the disability, and it was up to the rehabilitation therapist to "fix" or reduce the disability. Yet, "for occupational therapy, the very nature of the problem was not the disability, but the occupational performance of the person with the disability" (Friedland, 1998, p. 373). In response to the demands of World War II, the profession began trading crafts for functional occupations such as work-related tasks as the therapeutic medium when treating individuals with physical disabilities (Schwartz, 1998). The profession maintained its autonomy through increasing the standards of occupational therapy schools and ensuring that the directors of these programs and clinical training were qualified occupational therapists (Colman, 1992).

Although the rehabilitation movement provided new opportunities for occupational therapy, the literature indicates that an awkward alliance exists between occupational therapy and rehabilitation therapy. According to Friedland (1998), the professions' core concepts began to erode after World War II, when the development of rehabilitation and physical medicine occurred. Therefore, occupational therapy's core values conflicted with the paradigm of rehabilitation. This may partly explain the identity problems that occupational therapists experience today. The role of occupational therapy went from a focus on occupation as a means to good health and well-being to exercising a disabled body part during an activity to increase strength, range of motion, and motor skills. To compete with the status of physical therapy, "the physical aspects of treatment gained prominence over psychological concerns" (Friedland, 1998).

Recently, just as the World Health Organization's (WHO's) concept of health has been expanded to include more than the absence of disease or impairment, so too has the concept of rehabilitation been broadened to include some occupational therapy core concepts, such as promoting a fulfilling and productive life and social integration to ensure a successful rehabilitation outcome. These are unique skills of the occupational therapy profession. All occupational therapists and occupational therapy assistants need to return to the use of occupation to meet the client's goals and to proclaim the uniqueness of occupational therapy so the future of the profession will be preserved. This process of returning to our roots has begun with occupational therapy leaders such as those on the Practice Framework Committee at Cardinal Hill Rehabilitation Hospital by sharing our documentation.

Cardinal Hill Healthcare System

Cardinal Hill Rehabilitation Hospital (CHRH) began in 1950 with a 50-bed convalescent center serving Kentucky children with physical disabilities. Soon after, the Kentucky Crippled Children's Commission moved into the hospital to provide outpatient care for children. In 1952, ground was broken to create a nursery school that would provide education, recreation, and therapy treatment for children with cerebral palsy. Over time, the need for adult care increased, and the hospital was expanded to provide services for individuals following a cerebrovascular accident, spinal cord injury, traumatic brain injury, amputation, neurological condition, or pulmonary disorders. The expansion of all the programs led the hospital to become a part of the Easter Seals Society of Kentucky.

Today, Cardinal Hill Healthcare System (CHHS) consists of two inpatient hospitals. The main hospital specializes in the treatment of spinal cord injury, brain injury, stroke, multiple sclerosis, and other disabling conditions for people of all ages. The program includes a 108-bed inpatient facility, specialty therapy gyms, an indoor therapeutic swimming pool, a recreation center, a cafeteria, a gift shop, and a 4,000-square-ft. conference center. Cardinal Hill Specialty Hospital, a long-term acute care hospital in Ft. Thomas, Kentucky, has 35 beds. There are three outpatient programs, with the largest being at the main hospital in Lexington. The outpatient program shares all the hospital amenities; in addition, there is a fitness center, sensory integration gym, and state-of-the-art equipment. Other outpatient centers are in Louisville and Covington, both specializing in pediatric outpatient care. Camp Kysoc (*Keep Your Sight on Challenge*) in Carrolton provides camp experiences to individuals throughout the summers. In 2004, CHRH opened a home health division called Cardinal Hill Home Care, and in the one year since, 335 clients have been served in the nearby counties.

The mission of all of the facilities is to provide benchmark physical rehabilitation services while treating more than 6,000 people in Kentucky each year, representing all of the counties in the state (CHRH, 2000). Individuals come to the facilities from every county in Kentucky. An affiliation with the University of Kentucky medical school enables staff and clients to participate in research and teaching and to access the latest technology, which results in improved client care. CHRH is accredited by the Commission on the Accreditation of Rehabilitation Facilities.

CHHS has a rich heritage of 55 years of providing services and partnering with groups and institutions in the community. The facilities have a strong bond with the academic institutions in Kentucky, especially the Occupational Therapy Department at Eastern Kentucky University. The vision of the occupational therapy program at CHHS is to offer client-centered, evidence-based practice and to continually challenge the occupational therapists to apply theories into practice.

Occupational Therapy at Cardinal Hill

In the 1990s, the Cardinal Hill Occupational Therapy Department incorporated the *Uniform Terminology for Occupational Therapy–Third Edition* (*UT–III*; American Occupational Therapy Association [AOTA], 1994) in all its documentation and practiced within its guidelines. The therapists embraced the terminology, as it gave them boundaries to their practice, and they became comfortable talking about occupational therapy. They used theories to support the terminology for intervention and presented our documentation at professional conferences. As much as the CHHS occupational therapists liked *UT–III*, it somewhat limited the continuum of care for clients as compared to the *Practice Framework*. However, in the fall of 1998, AOTA's Commission on Practice began an extensive review process to solicit input from all levels of the occupational therapy profession with respect to the need for another revision of *UT–III* (AOTA, 2002). As changes occurred in the profession, a new document was developed by the commission based on feedback from occupational therapists and occupational therapy assistants who wanted a focus on occupation as the core of the profession (Harvison, 2003). This new document became the *Occupational Therapy Practice Framework: Domain and Process* (AOTA, 2002).

About This Book

The core authors felt a strong commitment to integrating the *Practice Framework* into practice at the Cardinal Hill Rehabilitation Hospital. Our intent was to create this book to serve as an example of how the *Practice Framework* can be used effectively in practice.

—Camille Skubik-Peplaski, MS, OTR/L, BCP;
Chasity Paris, MS, OTR/L;
Dana Rae Collins Boyle, OTR/L; and
Amy Culpert, OTR/L
Therapists, Cardinal Hill Healthcare Systems
Lexington, Kentucky

Acknowledgments

We extend special thanks to all the occupational therapists at Cardinal Hill Healthcare System for their support and feedback during this transition process and their commitment to providing benchmark services. We also thank Stephen Skubik-Peplaski and Courtney Williams, OTR/L, ATC, for their software support and knowledge.

Contributors

Contributing Authors to the Analysis, Profile, Protocols, and Intervention Plans—
 Marilyn Collins, OTR/L
 Laurie Nichols, OTR/L
 Linda Clark, OTR/L
 Kim Reninger, OTR/L
 Stacy Grider, OTR/L
 Linda Freudenberger, OTR/L
 Dan Hudson, OTR/L

Contributing Authors to the Pediatric Analysis and Protocol—
 Ariane Mongeau, OTR/L
 Courtney Williams, OTR/L
 Emily Rone, OTR/L
 Rebecca Johnson, MOT, OT/L
 Kim Ball, OTR/L
 Karen Summers, OTR/L
 Sally Lumm, OTR/L

All the occupational therapists are from the Cardinal Hill Healthcare System,
Lexington, Kentucky.

Contributions also were made by
 Anne Blakeney, PhD, OTR, FAOTA, Eastern Kentucky University, Richmond

Moving From *Uniform Terminology* to the *Practice Framework* at Cardinal Hill Healthcare System

Making the Transition

In early 2002, many occupational therapists at Cardinal Hill Healthcare System (CHHS) became familiar with the *Occupational Therapy Practice Framework: Domain and Process* (American Occupational Therapy Association [AOTA], 2002; see Appendix K) as it was evolving into practice, and we followed its progression. Later that year, a core group of therapists volunteered to explore integrating the *Framework* into our documentation. The transition began officially as we named our group the Practice Framework Committee. The occupational therapy practice coordinator, who is responsible for ensuring ethical and competent practice at our facility, led the committee. The committee first spent weeks together learning and studying the *Framework*. Previously, all of our documentation was rooted in the *Uniform Terminology for Occupational Therapy–Third Edition* (AOTA, 1994), and learning a new process was complicated and overwhelming. The committee encountered many roadblocks along the way, especially finding a starting point. We found that the therapists needed to shift from a component-based, therapist-driven focus to an occupation-based and client-centered focus. This transition was difficult at times but necessary as the *Framework* was in alignment with the World Health Organization's (WHO's) *International Classification of Functioning, Disability, and Health* (WHO, 2001). Initially the committee brainstormed and set the following objectives:

- Become competent in the use of the *Occupational Therapy Practice Framework* to guide occupation-based practice
- Develop a new occupational therapy evaluation and intervention plan in alignment with the *Framework*
- Increase all occupational therapists' knowledge of the *Framework* and use of the new evaluation and intervention plan
- Change the practice of occupational therapy within CHHS from a focus on clients' deficits to client-centered occupationally based practice.

During the process, the committee contacted the Kentucky Occupational Therapy Association; AOTA; and our nearby academic institution, Eastern Kentucky University. We also posted questions on an AOTA listserv but did not receive any feedback regarding written documentation using the *Framework*. Staff at AOTA were very helpful in providing feedback once the committee had written something. The professors at Eastern Kentucky University were knowledgeable in teaching the *Framework*'s content and incorporating the *Framework* into student assignments; however, they had limited recommendations for application to evaluations and intervention plans. The committee did contribute to the June 2003 *Administration and Management Special Interest Section Quarterly* by sharing how our facility was embracing the *Framework* (Gentile, 2003). Difficulty getting assistance did not hinder the committee as we continued to learn about the *Framework* and apply the concepts as we taught our peers through in-services, discussion groups, and student assignments. Learning about the *Framework* and creating all our documentation took about 1 year. After using our analysis and profile for 6 months, we began to receive requests from other professionals on how we implemented the *Framework,* and we continue to receive requests.

The CHHS administration often wondered why the committee's process was taking so long as we kept talking about changing. No one understood the large scope of the problem we were addressing. Hospital administration officials thought we should be able to make an easier transition, and they were concerned that we would stress the occupational therapy staff. Two members of senior management happened to be occupational therapists; this was very valuable, as they understood the need to shift our focus away from a medical model and embrace occupation.

Once the main hospital, including the adult and pediatric outpatient units, started using the new documentation, we ventured out to share it with our two other outpatient facilities. Resistance occurred in all settings, as the occupational therapists wanted to see how the evaluation and intervention plan worked before they tried it. The therapists resisted learning the new concepts that would expand their thought processes. Understanding this resistance phenomenon was made easier because of the information we had gained from the literature review. Therefore, the initial use of the evaluation was slow and tedious but, with time, all the staff began to use it.

Transition Process as Occupational Adaptation

Reflecting back, we now realize that occupational adaptation theory best describes both the process through which the committee went when it was creating the new evaluation and how our evaluation aligns with the *Framework*. Occupational adaptation theory offers the occupational therapy profession a discipline-specific theory of change. The three basic elements of the occupational adaptation process are (a) the person, (b) the occupational environment, and (c) the interaction between the two as they come together in occupation (Schkade & Shultz, 1992). This holistic approach facilitates clients' internal adaptation process to perform meaningful occupations with relative mastery or increased "efficiency, effectiveness, and satisfaction" (p. 830). Occupational adaptation facilitates the success in a client's desire for mastery of any chosen occupation (i.e., occupational therapy at CHHS; Schkade & Shultz, 1992). According to occupational adaptation theory, change occurs when the desire for mastery within a person and the demand for mastery from the environment create a press for mastery in response to an occupational challenge. The challenge for the occupational therapists at CHHS was using the *Framework* and a new occupational therapy evaluation.

In reaction to the press for mastery, the person generates an "adaptive response" to produce an occupational response (Schkade & Shultz, 1992, p. 832). The person then evaluates the occupational response on the basis of the perception of relative mastery and finally integrates the response to the occupational challenge into his or her adaptive repertoire. The outcome of this process is a change in occupational functioning that results in "one of three states: occupational adaptation, homeostasis, or occupational dysfunction" (p. 835). A person achieves a state of occupational adaptation when the occupational response is incorporated into his or her repertoire of adaptive responses and he or she generalizes or applies the responses to future occupational challenges. Difficulty in achieving occupational adaptation occurs when "those persons whose adaptive response evaluation and adaptive response integration subprocess are functioning marginally . . . as opposed to those with well-functioning subprocesses" (p. 836). Difficulty with achieving occupational adaptation was most apparent among the occupational therapists at Cardinal Hill Rehabilitation Hospital during the transition to the use of a new evaluation, as evidenced by their frustration with trying to use a holistic occupation-based tool with a medical model focus.

On the basis of our commitment to forge ahead and be a benchmark facility, we embraced the *Framework*'s concepts and empowered others with constant support and enthusiasm. Change was evident in environmental shifts such as the purchase of more occupation-based supplies, including gardening supplies, poker games and chips, bocce ball games, brooms and cleaning equipment, and fishing equipment. The Level II fieldwork students contributed by creating occupation-based activities, including motors and mechanical parts, tool benches, and home repair kits. The process took time, compromise, and patience, but in the end, client-centered practice was evident, and occupational adaptation was achieved among both occupational therapists and clients.

Using the *Framework* in Evaluation

On the basis of the committee's understanding of the *Occupational Therapy Practice Framework: Domain and Process* (American Occupational Therapy Association [AOTA], 2002; see Appendix K), we felt that the evaluation should consist of two parts: (a) the Cardinal Hill Healthcare System Occupational Profile (see Appendix A) and (b) the Cardinal Hill Healthcare System Occupational Analysis (see Appendix B). The committee struggled with how to capture the dynamic process of the *Framework* into a written evaluation form. In looking at the six categories outlined in the domain of practice (performance in areas of occupation, performance skills, client factors, context, activity demands, and performance patterns), the committee decided that the Occupational Profile would best represent the client's performance patterns, contexts, and activity demands. The performance in areas of occupation, skills, and client factors would be covered in the Occupational Analysis. It was understood that all aspects of the domains are considered in the profile and analysis as they relate to the client. Figure 2.1 is adapted from the *Framework* so that one can more easily visualize how the committee broke down the *Framework* to use in evaluation.

Cardinal Hill Healthcare System Occupational Profile

The committee first wrote the Occupational Profile (see Figure 2.2). During this process, we focused on gaining information on the client's occupational history, values, roles, interests, habits, needs, and experiences. The ultimate goal of the profile was to provide client-centered therapy by understanding the client's perspective of the occupations that he or she wanted or needed to perform to participate in life. The committee formulated questions by reading suggestions from the *Framework* that related to the three domains of interest previously mentioned.

In accordance with the *Framework*'s suggestion of using theories and frames of references to guide reasoning, the committee decided to draw conceptually from the Canadian Model of Occupational Performance (COPM; Law et al., 1994). The COPM has clients identify occupations according to priority and rate levels of satisfaction in occupational performance. Therefore, we created an area on the evaluation form within the Occupational Profile titled "Occupations Client Wants/Needs to Resume" (see Figure 2.3). It is here that clients identify five areas of occupation during the initial evaluation that they wish to pursue

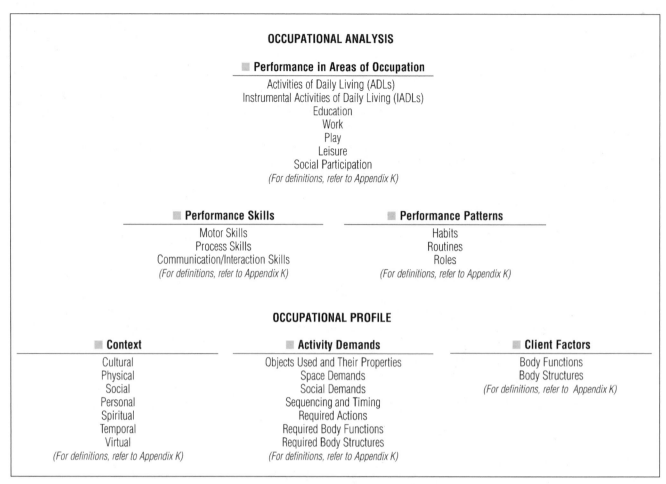

Figure 2.1. Domain of occupational therapy, as broken down for the Cardinal Hill Healthcare System.
From "Occupational therapy practice framework: Domain and process," by the American Occupational Therapy Association, 2002, *American Journal of Occupational Therapy, 56*, p. 611.
Copyright © 2002 by the American Occupational Therapy Association. Adapted with permission.

during occupational therapy intervention. At discharge, if appropriate, the client rates his or her level of satisfaction in performing these occupations on a scale of 1 through 10, with 1 being *Not Satisfied* and 10 being *Very Satisfied*.

An interesting aspect of the Occupational Profile was the idea that the client could control his or her intervention plan. For example, individuals could name any occupation that they wanted to resume or learn. They did not have to be constrained to only basic self-care and activities of daily living (ADLs). Although we knew that some occupations chosen may not be realistic or feasible at this stage and time in some clients' rehabilitation process, the occupational therapists would still be able to use preparatory activities, as suggested by the *Framework,* to facilitate the client's progress toward resuming his or her chosen occupations.

The importance of the Occupational Profile was never underestimated, as the committee knew its information would guide the occupational therapists' intervention planning and process. It was predicted that it would ultimately result in increased client satisfaction, participation, and goal attainment. Therefore, the committee determined that if the client were cognitively unable to participate in the profile, then family members or caregivers would be asked to supply information.

1. Client lives ☐ alone ☐ with _____ in a ☐ house ☐ trailer ☐ apt. with _____ steps to enter ☐ R ☐ L handrail; _____ stories; _____ steps inside home. _____

2. Client's discharge environment, resources, and available adaptive equipment: _____

3. Prior to this hospitalization, the client was ☐ I ☐ min ☐ mod in ADLs and ☐ I ☐ min ☐ mod in IADLs. Client needed assistance with

4. A typical day consists of: wake-up time _____ ☐ a.m. ☐ p.m.; ☐ volunteer ☐ work; bedtime _____ ☐ a.m. ☐ p.m.

5. What activities do you participate in for fun and how often? _____

6. How do you learn best? (In rehab you will be learning new things. Do you learn best by reading, watching a video?) _____

7. How familiar are you with technology? _____

8. What motivates you to improve? _____

9. How are you coping with your current status? _____

Figure 2.2. Cardinal Hill Healthcare System Occupational Profile, Questions 1–9.
Note. R/L = right/left; I = independent; min = minimum; mod = moderate; ADLs = activities of daily living; IADLs = instrumental activities of daily living.

Cardinal Hill Occupational Analysis

The next challenge was the creation of the Occupational Analysis. We began writing the analysis with a focus on performance in areas of occupation. Specific emphasis was placed on assessing basic activities of daily living (BADLs) to meet both our facility's requirements and reimbursement requirements. The BADLs were assessed using the Functional

Initial Comments	Discharge Comments
List 5 occupations you want/need to resume	Satisfaction in resuming your roles
1.	
2.	
3.	
4.	
5.	

Figure 2.3. Bottom section of Cardinal Hill Healthcare System Occupational Profile.

Independence Measure (FIM; Uniform Data System for Medical Rehabilitation, 1997), which also is a facility requirement. However, we did not allow these requirements to prevent us from analyzing other areas of occupation as identified in the Occupational Profile. The BADL and instrumental activities of daily living (IADLs) portion of the analysis can be seen in Figure 2.4. It is important to note that certain terms were chosen to respect other disciplines and their roles in the rehabilitation team at CHHS.

Next, the committee examined performance skills, activity demands, and client factors that were most applicable to our practice setting, with comment sections available for

Initial Comments		Discharge Comments
	Basic ADLs	
	Eating	
	Grooming	
	Bathing	
	E/W/S Dressing UB E/W/S	
	E/W/S Dressing LB E/W/S	
	Toilet TX	
	Tub/Shower TX	
	Problem Solving	
	Memory	
	Comments	
	Instrumental ADLs	
	Community Mobility	
	Health Management	
	Home Management	
	Financial Management	
	Leisure	
	Safety	
	Comments	

Figure 2.4. Cardinal Hill Healthcare System Occupational Analysis.
Note. ADLs = activities of daily living; E/W/S = edge of bed/wheelchair/supine; UB = upper body; LB = lower body; TX = transfer.

additional observations. The committee decided to evaluate neuromusculoskeletal and movement-related functions (e.g., strength, muscle tone, range of motion, alignment, reflexes) of task performance. A functional movement grid to replace the traditional range-of-motion and manual muscle testing grid was one of the most instrumental changes the committee incorporated into the evaluation. The committee struggled with creating an appropriate layout with specific functional tasks that would demonstrate quality of movement versus movement deficits. The movement function section, including the grid, is depicted in Figure 2.5.

The pivotal moment in the design and layout of the functional movement grid occurred when one of the committee members awoke at 3:00 a.m. with an epiphany. She realized that the committee had been trying to make the functional movement grid too objective. The committee decided to focus on assessing the client's performance of six functional tasks (place can on shelf, retrieve item from floor, screw lid on jar, comb back of head, write name, and lift grocery bag) and within the grid make notes about the quality of movement, strength and effort, involuntary movements, muscle tone, range of motion, reflexes, and so on. The committee drew from the work of Taub and Wolf's (1997) constraint-induced movement therapy and the Arm Motor Activity Test (Taub, Crago, & McCulloch, 1997) in writing the protocol for quality of movement within the functional movement grid.

Another significant change from the old evaluation to the new one was based on feedback from AOTA's Program Director of Evidence-Based Practice, Deborah Lieberman, MHSA, OTR/L, FAOTA. She was very interested in our project from the beginning and was able to give feedback after we provided copies of our analysis and profile and information about our facility. She believed that our evaluation needed to be able to reflect the benefit of occupational

Initial Comments		Discharge Comments
	Movement Function	
	Sitting—Static/Dynamic	
	Standing—Static/Dynamic	
	Place can on shelf	
	Retrieve item from floor	
	Screw lid on jar	
	Comb back of head	
	Write name	
	Lift grocery bag	
	Comments	

Figure 2.5. Movement function section of the Cardinal Hill Healthcare System Occupational Analysis.

therapy services and how the client would generalize the skills he or she learned in therapy to the home environment. Therefore, a narrative question at the end of the analysis was added.

The initial evaluation question asks "How do the risks interfere with participation in occupation?" (see Figure 2.6). This question requires the occupational therapist to summarize the client's specific areas of occupation at risk for resumption of roles and to briefly describe the most significant factors compromising participation in occupations. This narrative was included to justify the client's need for occupational therapy. At discharge, the narrative question on the evaluation is "How has occupational therapy facilitated participation in occupation in client's environment?" This is where the therapist provides a summary of occupational therapy interventions and education used to facilitate the client's safe and independent transition to the discharge environment. This information demonstrates the need for a skilled service so a client can receive occupational therapy services at initial assessment and understand the benefits of our services at discharge.

It was difficult to stay motivated during this year-long process, especially when asked to defend our desire to focus on the clients and what they need to engage in occupation. Sometimes it seemed too much to tackle. However, the committee members tried to keep each other motivated by continually revisiting the importance of this project and what we hoped it would do for our practice. We also stayed motivated by setting deadlines along the way and delegating some different areas of the evaluation to specific committee members on the basis of their personal interests and areas of expertise. This helped us accomplish small goals every week. Sections that were worked on individually were then presented, discussed, and further developed at our weekly meetings. The completion of some sections was more gratifying than others.

When we finished the Occupational Profile, we knew we could handle the Occupational Analysis. Moving through the BADLs and IADLs and finally coming to an agreement on what items would be listed and what items were to be covered under comments was an accomplishment, but the biggest satisfaction was when we conceptualized the movement function grid. We knew it was innovative and challenging and that some therapists would

How do the risks interfere with participation in occupation?	How has occupational therapy facilitated participation in occupation in client's environment?

Figure 2.6. Narrative questions added at the end of the Cardinal Hill Healthcare System Occupational Analysis.

have a hard time shifting to the new concepts, but it turned out to show what we wanted: the impact of barriers on movement for occupation. The rest of the evaluation came together after that. The final paragraphs were written, and we then added the information that had to be gathered at discharge. Watching the progress was fascinating, revitalizing, and affirming, and it strengthened our commitment to the profession and the clients we serve.

Intervention Plan

When the Occupational Profile and Occupational Analysis were completed, we began working on the intervention plan (see Appendixes C and D). The first dilemma we faced was trying to identify which new *Framework* words to use to describe the risks and occupations so that reimbursement sources would recognize and pay for them (e.g., energy for task, fluidity of movement). We also wanted a checklist format so that the issues that affected each client could be quickly identified. We knew that we had to include short- and long-term goals, client strengths, plan of care, occupational therapy diagnosis, duration, precautions, and professional signatures. Once again, we started splitting up the areas identified by the *Framework* and listing occupations in which the client participated. As we began to understand the *Framework* more thoroughly, we knew we needed to include an assessment of the client's satisfaction in his or her ability to participate in his or her chosen occupations. The next section identified the risks that interfered with participation. We used *Framework* terminology to describe each of these categories and listed the options below each heading. A breakthrough occurred when we visualized client strengths or weaknesses as contextual influences that affect performance and intervention planning.

When we began discussing goals, we realized that we had to write two different forms of the intervention plan because of the payment focus based on the FIM for inpatient clients. We chose 15 prewritten long-term goals covering all BADLs and some IADLs and 2 open goals for the inpatient intervention plan. The open narrative goals allow for more flexibility and the choosing of goals specific to client occupations. The short-term goals are specifically written for each client.

Another intervention plan was created for use with outpatients because of the variety of clients, including pediatric. Because of this, short- and long-term goals were left open-ended so they could be specifically tailored to each client. The intervention plan focused on the approaches that would be used to meet the goals and resolve the risks for participation in occupation. We worked to include modalities and different interventions (e.g., hippotherapy, aquatics) that therapy would entail. The intervention plan includes duration and frequency, which is critical because reimbursement sources want specific information on the length of the admission and the times per week or day a client will be seen by the therapist. The medical diagnosis is included as well as the occupational therapy diagnosis. It is important that these diagnoses are not the same, as occupational therapists cannot provide a medical diagnosis but can diagnose occupational performance issues. Signature and date conclude the treatment plan.

When we finished, we realized that once a client had identified on the Occupational Profile the areas he or she wanted to resume or learn, it became easy to write client goals on the intervention plan. This further solidified a client-centered approach to intervention and strengthened our partnership with the client.

Protocols

After all the parts of the evaluation were written, the committee found that we needed to write directions on how to use it. Again, we delegated parts to committee members, and each one started with the *Framework* definitions to shape their sections. They then created specific questions for each section as to how an occupational therapist would be able to obtain the information needed from the client. The definitions, observations, and evaluation questions were combined to create a long protocol for adults (see Appendix E). A short protocol for adults was created and included the evaluation questions and observations (see Appendix F). At first, both protocols were cumbersome, and therapists found it difficult to work through them. With time, they learned the new definitions and how to use the evaluation questions. We had occupational therapy students make shortened versions of the protocols (cue sheets) so that the occupational analysis would be more time efficient. We found that each of the programs in the hospital required a different type of modified cue sheet because different sections of the evaluation are stressed with different diagnoses (e.g., a client with traumatic brain injury requires more specific cognitive assessments than a client who has had a knee replacement).

Pediatric Analysis of Occupational Performance

Pediatric Occupational Therapy Evaluation

The Cardinal Hill Healthcare System Protocol for Pediatric Occupational Therapy Evaluation (see Appendix G) was adapted from the original profile by the pediatric staff at Cardinal Hill Rehabilitation Hospital. It was designed to reflect how the child's age may affect his or her roles, performance patterns, contexts, and activity demands. The protocol that was developed by the core committee related to the client's assistance level before and after admission to the hospital. Although this facility treats clients who have been referred after an injury, the majority of the pediatric clients seen at this facility are referred because of a condition acquired at birth. Therefore, Question 3 on the original profile regarding status before admission was eliminated from the pediatric profile.

The most important part of the profile involves the family and the child identifying and prioritizing the five occupations they want addressed in therapy (see Figure 2.3). Parents establish occupational goals for children who are very young or cognitively unable to establish their own goals. However, the majority of children are encouraged to participate in setting their own occupational priorities. At discharge, the family and child's level of satisfaction in occupational goals is indicated.

Pediatric Occupational Profile

The Cardinal Hill Healthcare System Occupational Profile (see Appendix H) was developed on the basis of the areas of occupation that pertain to children. These include BADLs, IADLs, education, play/leisure, and social participation. Performance skills and patterns, activity demands, and client factors within the areas of occupation are evaluated with standardized tests, normed tests, child/parent interview, observation of occupational performance, or some combination of these. The pediatric occupational therapy team included standardized test results as a part of the evaluation to provide a baseline for the child's functional status. These test results also are used by reimbursement sources, families, teachers, and doctors to understand the child's occupational performance level. The pediatric occupational therapy team determined that the standardized tests complemented the child/parent interview and direct observation of performance to provide a well-rounded picture of the child's performance level.

The entire pediatric occupational therapy team participated in the development of the evaluation to encourage a user-friendly tool that would be embraced by the whole team. We began with the outline of the original evaluation and quickly decided that it did not meet all the specific needs of pediatric clients. The original evaluation did not provide room for standardized test results, and the evaluation protocol referred to adult occupations only. All of the pediatric occupational therapists met as a team to discuss a vision of a new pediatric occupational therapy evaluation based on the *Framework*. The protocol proved to be quite an undertaking because it needed to reflect the many developmental levels seen in clients of various ages. The evaluation and protocol was divided among the pediatric occupational therapists, who worked on the parts individually. The pediatric team met on several subsequent occasions to discuss progress and to put all the pieces together.

Using the Cardinal Hill Occupational Participation Process: Examples of Documentation

To assist readers in the application of the *Framework* in practice, this chapter includes samples of documentation for clients with the following diagnoses:

- Lumbar 1 fracture, spinal cord injury (Figures 3.1–3.3; case of J. R.)
- Cerebral vascular accident (Figures 3.4–3.6; case of C. G.)
- Closed head injury (Figures 3.7–3.9; case of K. H.)
- Dyspraxia (Figures 3.10–3.12; case of C. C.).

These examples are a compilation of therapists' experiences treating a variety of diagnoses. They do not represent specific clients at Cardinal Hill Healthcare System.

Cardinal Hill Healthcare System
Occupational Profile (Adult)

Client Name: _J. R._   Client #: _____ DOB: _11-1-76_

Initial Date: _2-1-05_   Discharge Date: _3-3-05_

Diagnosis: _L1 fracture_

Precautions: _TLSO when head of bed is > 30 degrees, no hip flexion > 90 degrees, Ted hose, abdominal binder_

1. Client lives ☑with ☐ alone _husband, 5-year-old son and 5-week-old daughter_ in a ☑house ☐ trailer ☐ apt. with __2__ steps to enter ☐ R/ ☐ L handrail; __2__ stories; _____ steps inside home. _____

2. Client's discharge environment, resources, and available adaptive equipment: _2-tub/shower combos and 2 standard commodes with no adaptations._

3. Prior to this hospitalization, the client was ☑I ☐ min ☐ mod in BADLs and ☑I ☐ min ☐ mod in IADLs. Client needed assistance with _complex home repairs._

4. A typical day consists of: wake up time __6:00__ ☑a.m. ☐ p.m.; ☐ volunteer ☐ work; bedtime __11:00__ ☐ a.m. ☑p.m.
   Monday through Friday, the client would get up and get son ready for school and fix breakfast, then she would take along the baby when she took her son to school. At noon she would pick her son up from school and fix lunch for him. In the afternoon she spent time housecleaning and playing with her children. Then she would fix dinner and then bathe her children before putting them to bed, which was usually around 8:00 pm. Lastly, she would spend time with her husband. On the weekends she spent time with her husband and children by attending her son's ballgames or watching movies together. She and her family attended church on Sundays.

5. What activities do you participate in for fun and how often? _Attend son's weekly ballgames, church activities on Wednesday nights, go out to eat with friends once a month_

6. How do you learn best? (In rehab you will be learning new things. Do you learn best by reading, watching a video?) _____ _"By watching a demonstration and then practicing it over and over"_

7. How familiar are you with technology? _I can use the word processor and Internet fairly well_

8. What motivates you to improve? _I want to be able to take care of myself and my family again_

9. How are you coping with your current status? _I take it one day at a time…I still cry and feel depressed when I think about my life sometimes_

Initial Comments   **Discharge Comments**

List 5 occupations you want/need to resume	Satisfaction in resuming your roles
Play with children	_Satisfied 6/10_
Cook for family	_Satisfied 6/10_
Dress by myself	_Satisfied 8/10_
Bathe myself	_Satisfied 7/10_
Church activities	_Satisfied 9/10_

Therapist's Signature _____ Date _____ Therapist's Signature _____ Date

Figure 3.1. Cardinal Hill Healthcare System Occupational Profile (Adult): Case of J. R.
Note. L1 = Lumbar 1; TLSO = thoracic lumbar sacral orthotic; I = independent; min = minimum; mod = moderate; R/L = right/left; BADLs = basic activities of daily living; IADLs = instrumental activities of daily living.

Cardinal Hill Healthcare System
Occupational Analysis (Adult)

Client Name: _J. R._ Client #: _____ DOB: _11-1-76_

Initial Date: _2-1-05_ Discharge Date: _3-5-05_

Diagnosis: _Lumbar 1 fracture_

Precautions: _Thoracic Lumbar Sacral Orthotic (TLSO) on when head of bed > 30 degrees, abdominal binder, Ted hose, no hip flexion > 90 degrees_

Occupational Analysis:

Initial Comments	**Basic ADLs**	**Discharge Comments**
Independent with tray setup	Eating	Independent with tray setup
Min A w/c level at sink	Grooming	Independent w/c level at sink
Max A with sponge bath	Bathing	Min A using long-handled sponge
Min A with pullover shirt	E/W/**S** Dressing UB E/W/**S**	Setup to donn TLSO
Dependent – client does < 25%	E/W/**S** Dressing LB E/W/**S**	Setup using adaptive equipment
Dependent – client does < 25%	Toilet TX	Standby assist using sliding board
Dependent – client does < 25%	Tub/Shower TX	Min A using sliding board to padded transfer tub bench with cutout
>10% vc for complex tasks	Problem Solving	Independent for complex tasks
Independent for daily routine	Memory	Independent for daily routine
Requires meds to sleep	Comments	No meds to sleep at night

Figure 3.2. Cardinal Hill Healthcare System Analysis (Adult): Case of J. R.

(continued)

17

Client Name: _J. R._ _____ Client #: _____

Initial Comments   **Discharge Comments**

Prior to injury client:	**Instrumental ADLs**	**At home client will:**
Drove minivan independently	Community Mobility	_Be dependent on family_
Was independent with med routine	Health Management	_Be independent with med routine_
Dusted, mopped, cooked, vacuumed	Home Management	_Hire help to clean house 1x wk_
Organized budget and paid bills	Financial Management	_Balance budget/pay bills with husband_
Read, watched movies, took long walks	Leisure	_Read, watch movies_
Demonstrated appropriate 911 response	Safety	_Demonstrate appropriate 911 response_
Fed and cared for family dog	Comments	_Care for dog with assist from husband_
	Movement Function	
Fair/Poor	Sitting—Static/Dynamic	_Good/Good_
_N/A_	Standing—Static/Dynamic	_N/A_
L1 fracture	Joint Stability and Skeletal Mobility	_L1 fracture_

Figure 3.2. Cardinal Hill Healthcare System Occupational Analysis (Adult): Case of J. R. _(continued)._

Client Name: _J. R._____ Client #: _____

Initial Comments   **Discharge Comments**

Initial Comments		Discharge Comments
Able to perform with both UEs, but has to stabilize self with opposing arm to prevent loss of balance	Place can on shelf	*Able to perform with both UEs without having to stabilize self*
Unable with either UE secondary to hip precautions	Retrieve item from floor	*Able with both UEs using a reacher*
Able with RUE, uses LUE as a stabilizer	Screw lid on jar	*Able with RUE, uses LUE as a stabilizer*
Able with both UEs	Comb back of head	*Able with both UEs*
Able with R hand	Write name	*Able with R hand*
Able with both UEs from waist to head level	Lift grocery bag	*Able with both UEs from waist to head level*
Client has WNL ROM and MMT of both UEs in order to participate in BADLs/IADLs	Comments	*Client has WNL ROM and MMT of both UEs in order to participate in BADLs/IADLs*

Figure 3.2. Cardinal Hill Healthcare System Occupational Analysis (Adult): Case of J. R. *(continued)*.

(continued)

Client Name: _J. R._ _____ Client #: _____

Initial Comments   **Discharge Comments**

Initial Comments								Category	Discharge Comments							
Fair during a.m. BADLs								Energy for Task	*Good for a.m. BADLs*								
WFL for fmc, gmc, bilateral int.								Coordination	*WFL for a.m. BADLs*								
L	58#	13#	17#	R	60#	14#	17#	Grip Strength/Lateral Pinch lbs/3 Jaw Chuck	L	63#	13#	17#	R	63#	14#	17#	
WFL – gathers appropriate items								Knowledge/Organization of Task	*WFL*								
Impaired – needs assist to use AE or adaptive strategies to complete tasks efficiently and effectively								Adaptation/Praxis	*WFL – uses AE and adapted strategies appropriately*								
								Comments									
Good eye contact during conversation. Expresses anxiety and depression about being able to play with children.								**Social Interaction Skills**	*Cooperative and friendly, expresses excitement about getting back home to her family*								
								Cognitive & Affective									
Attends to multi-step ADLs								Level of Arousal/Attention	*Attends to multi-step ADLs*								
A & 0 x 4								Orientation	*A & 0 x 4*								
Motivated to be independent with BADL/IADLs								Energy and Drive	*Motivated to continue being as independent as possible at home*								

Figure 3.2. Cardinal Hill Healthcare System Occupational Analysis (Adult): Case of J. R. *(continued).*

Client Name: *J. R.* _____ Client #: _____

Initial Comments   **Discharge Comments**

Initial Comments		Discharge Comments
Performs routine tasks independently *Needs min A for nonroutine tasks*	**Higher Level Cognition**	*Independent with all nonroutine tasks*
Light tough, pain, and temp absent in dermatomes L2 and below	**Sensory**	*Same as initial evaluation*
No problems per client	**Visual**	*Same as initial evaluation*
Doubtful about regaining prior function	**Perception**	*Increased confidence in her independence with roles at home*
6 out of 10 in lower back	**Pain**	*3 out of 10 in lower back*
Back incision intact	**Skin Integrity**	*Staples in back have been removed*
Need education on appropriate pressure relief purpose and technique	Comments	*Client independently performs pressure relief*

	Pre	Post		Pre	Post		Pre	Post		Pre	Post		Pre	Post		Pre	Post
HR	65	68	O_2	99	99	RPD	1	2	HR	66	67	O_2	98	99	RPD	1	2

Information taken during a.m. BADLs	Comments	*Information taken during a.m. BADLs*

Figure 3.2. Cardinal Hill Healthcare System Occupational Analysis (Adult): Case of J. R. *(continued)*.

(continued)

Client Name: _J. R._ _____ Client #: _____

Initial Comments   **Discharge Comments**

How do the risks interfere with participation in occupation?

Client wants to return home to take care of self and family.
Client needs to increase independence in all ADLs using AE and
strategies. Also, client needs to increase UB strength, sitting
static/dynamic balance, and energy for task to complete desired
occupations.

How has occupational therapy facilitated participation in occupation
in client's environment?

Client now performs all ADLs with min A or better in order for
her to return home to family. Client uses AE that will be used
in home environment safely, and spouse demonstrates and
understands all training in these areas.

Equipment:

TBA

Equipment provided:

Reacher, leg lifter, long-handled sponge, cup holder. Ordered
client a padded transfer tub bench with cutout.

Goals met:

1–9

Goals not met:

Unable to complete tub transfers with SBA secondary to
decreased balance and safety

Number of visits:

N/A

ELOS:

3–4 weeks

Reason for discharge:
Maximum rehab potential met for inpatient stay

D/C recommendations/referrals:
Outpatient occupational therapy

_____ _____   _____ _____
Therapist's Signature   Date   Therapist's Signature   Date

Figure 3.2. Cardinal Hill Healthcare System Occupational Analysis (Adult): Case of J. R. *(continued).*

Note. ADLs = activities of daily living; Min = minimum; A = assistance; w/c = wheelchair; E/W/S = edge of bed/wheelchair/supine; UB = upper body; LB = lower body; donn = put on; TX = transfer; vc = verbal
cues; L1 = Lumbar 1; UE = upper extremity; RUE = right upper extremity; LUE = left upper extremity; R = right; WNL = within normal limits; ROM = range of motion; MMT = manual muscle test; BADLs = basic
activities of daily living; IADLs = instrumental activities of daily living; WFL = within functional limits; fmc = fine motor coordination; gmc = gross motor coordination; bilateral int. = bilateral integration; AE =
adaptive equipment; A & O x 4 = alert and oriented; L2 = Lumbar 2; HR = heart rate; O$_2$ = oxygen; RPD = rate of perceived dyspnea; ELOS = estimated length of stay; UB = upper body; SBA = standby assist;
D/C = discharge.

Cardinal Hill Healthcare System
Inpatient Intervention Plan

Client: *J. R.*   Client #: *12345-1*   DOB: *11/1/76*

Admit Date: *2/1/05*

Decreased satisfaction/ability to participate in the following occupations:

☑ Eating   ☑ Community Mobility   ☑ Shopping
☑ Grooming   ☑ Safety/Emergency Response   ☐ Education
☑ Bathing   ☐ Financial Management   ☐ Work
☑ Dressing   ☑ Health Management   ☑ Leisure/Play
☑ Toilet Transfer   ☑ Home Management   ☑ Functional Mobility
☐ Tub/Shower Transfer   ☑ Social Participation

Performance risks that interfere with participation in occupations:

☑ Problem Solving   ☐ Neuromuscular/Movement   ☑ Skin Integrity
☐ Memory   ☐ Oral Motor/Dysphagia   ☑ Pain
☐ Cognition   ☑ Mobility   ☑ Organization/Adaptability
☐ Posture   ☐ Coordination   ☐ Sensory Functions
☑ Energy/Endurance   ☑ Strength/Effort   ☐ Vision Functions
☑ Perception

Strengths (contextual influences): *motivated to be independent with BADLs*

Short-term goals: *Client will: 1. Participate in initial eval and goal setting.*
2. Dress lower body with moderate assistance using adaptive equipment in bed.
3. Prepare simple meal with minimal assistance using adaptive equipment.

Discharge Goals/Rehab Potential: Client will demonstrate:

☐ 1. Eating with *Independence* using _____
☑ 2. Grooming with *Independence at sink, wheelchair level* using _____ ☐ w/c level ☐ walker level ☐ standing
☑ 3. Bathing with *minimal assistance using adaptive equipment* using _____ ☐ sponge bath ☐ tub bath
☑ 4. Upper body dressing with *setup for TLSO at EOB* using _____ ☐ EOB ☐ w/c level ☐ supine
☑ 5. Lower body dressing with *setup and supervision at EOB* using _____ ☐ EOB ☐ w/c level ☐ supine
☑ 6. Toilet transfer with *SBA* using *sliding board to elevated commode with rails* ☐ w/c level ☐ walker level
☑ 7. Tub/shower transfer with *SBA* using *sliding board to transfer tub bench, wheelchair* ☐ w/c level ☐ walker level
☑ 8. Problem solving with *Independence for complex tasks*
☑ 9. Memory with *Independence for daily routines*
☑ 10. Light homemaking activities with *modified independence* using *wheelchair* ☐ w/c level ☐ walker level

Client/Family will:

☑ 11. Demonstrate knowledge to assist client with ADLs as needed
☑ 12. Perform home program with *setup* assistance
☑ 13. Participate in community outing with *minimal* assistance ☑ w/c level ☐ walker level
☑ 14. Demonstrate use of equipment with *supervision* assistance
☑ 15. Engage in leisure exploration and/or participation with *supervision*
☑ 16. *Demonstrate appropriate pressure relief techniques with independence.*
☐ 17. _____

Figure 3.3. Cardinal Hill Healthcare System Inpatient Intervention Plan: Case of J. R.

(continued)

Plan of Treatment/Education in:

☑ ADL	☐ Work/Productive Activities	☑ Psychosocial	☐ Positioning
☐ Neuromuscular Movement	☐ Cognitive Activities	☐ Sensory Activities	☐ Aquatics
☐ Skin/Edema	☐ Splinting/Casting	☑ Perceptual Tasks	☑ Leisure
☐ Modalities	☐ Oral Motor/Swallowing	☐ Re-Evaluation	☐ Co-Treat
☑ Adaptive Equipment	☑ D/C Planning	☐ Home Visit	☐ Other
☑ Home Program	☑ Client/Caregiver Education	☑ Home Safety/Equipment	

Frequency: *.5–1.5 hours, Mon–Sunday* Duration: *3–4 weeks*

Medical Diagnosis: *Lumbar 1 fracture*

OT Diagnosis: *decreased participation in BADL/IADLs and occupations*

Contraindications/Precautions: *TLSO on when head of bed > 30 degrees, abdominal binder, Ted hose, no hip flexion > 90 degrees*

I certify that occupational therapy services are necessary under a plan to be periodically reviewed by me and while the patient is under my care.

_____	_____	_____	_____
Date	Therapist's Signature	Accepted Date	Physician's Signature

Figure 3.3. Cardinal Hill Healthcare System Inpatient Intervention Plan: Case of J. R. *(continued)*.

Note. TLSO = thoracic lumbar sacral orthotic; EOB = edge of bed; w/c = wheelchair; SBA = standby assistance; ADLs = activities of daily living; BADLs = basic activities of daily living; IADLs = instrumental activities of daily living; UB = upper body; LB = lower body; D/C = discharge.

Cardinal Hill Healthcare System
Occupational Profile (Adult)

Client Name: *G. C.*   Client #: _____   DOB: *12-05-36*

Initial Date: *6-6-05*   Discharge Date: *7-1-05*

Diagnosis: *CVA with Left Hemiplegia*

Precautions: *Cardiac, fall precautions*

1. Client lives ☑ with ☐ alone *wife of 28 years* in a ☑ house ☐ trailer ☐ apt. with *1* steps to enter ☐ R/ ☐ L handrail; *2* stories; *14* steps inside home. *He has two children who live in the same community as well. Client's bedroom and shower/tub are located on the second floor.*

2. Client's discharge environment, resources, and available adaptive equipment: *Client plans to return home with his wife. He has no adaptive equipment. He has 2 tub/shower combos.*

3. Prior to this hospitalization, the client was ☑ I ☐ min ☐ mod in BADLs and ☑ I ☐ min ☐ mod in IADLs. Client needed assistance with *no occupations.*

4. A typical day consists of: wake up time *5:30* ☑ a.m. ☐ p.m.; ☐ volunteer ☐ work; bedtime *8:30* ☐ a.m. ☑ p.m. *Client begins his day by getting dressed and eating a small breakfast such as cereal. Since his retirement 10 years ago from an engineering firm, he spends lots of time working around the house. After breakfast he usually likes to assist his wife in cleaning up the house and work in the yard the rest of the morning. After eating lunch with his wife, he enjoys running errands or doing some woodwork in his garage. In the evenings, he has dinner with his wife, they often go out to eat, and they visit family or friends. He usually attends church on Sunday mornings.*

5. What activities do you participate in for fun and how often? *Woodworking (especially wood instruments), going out to eat, yard work*

6. How do you learn best? (In rehab you will be learning new things. Do you learn best by reading, watching a video?) *"I learn best through hands-on activities and practice."*

7. How familiar are you with technology? *Uses computer for e-mail and to research items of interest.*

8. What motivates you to improve? *The idea of getting back to being the same person I was before.*

9. How are you coping with your current status? *Not well; I've been depressed and anxious at times. Client was labile at times during evaluation. Client had a pulmonary embolism after his stroke and fears another episode.*

Initial Comments   **Discharge Comments**

List 5 occupations you want/need to resume	Satisfaction in resuming your roles
Going to the bathroom by myself	Satisfied; rates a 8/10 "since I still need supervision"
Walking upstairs and getting in my bed	Satisfied; did with his wife on day pass; rates 6/10
Dressing myself	Very satisfied; rates a 9/10
Bathing myself	Very Satisfied; rates a 9/10
Doing laundry	Satisfied; rates a 5/10 "I can help fold, but it's difficult"
Woodworking	Unsatisfied; rates a 2/10 "I can't do this very well"

Therapist's Signature   Date   Therapist's Signature   Date

Figure 3.4. Cardinal Hill Healthcare System Occupational Profile (Adult): Case of G. C.
Note. R/L = right/left; min = minimum; mod = moderate; CVA = cerebral vascular accident; I = independent; BADLs = basic activities of daily living; IADLs = instrumental activities of daily living.

Cardinal Hill Healthcare System
Occupational Analysis (Adult)

Client Name: *G. C.* Client #: ___ DOB: *12-05-36*

Initial Date: *6-6-05* Discharge Date: *7-1-05*

Diagnosis: *CVA with Left Hemiplegia*

Precautions: *Cardiac, fall precautions*

Occupational Analysis:

Initial Comments   **Discharge Comments**

Initial Comments	Basic ADLs	Discharge Comments
5 setup/supervision to open containers	Eating	*5 setup/supervision*
4 minimal assistance to wash left hand	Grooming	*7 independent; w/c level*
4 moderate assistance; washed 5/10 parts	Bathing	*5 setup/supervision*
3 moderate assistance; did 50%; EOB	E/W/S Dressing UB E/W/S	*5 setup/supervision; EOB*
2 maximum assistance; did < 50%; w/c level	E/**W**/S Dressing LB E/W/S	*5 setup/supervision; EOB*
4 minimum assistance, stand–pivot to elevated commode with rails	Toilet TX	*5 standby assist; supervision; stand–pivot to elevated toilet seat with rails*
3 moderate assistance, stand–pivot to shower with chair	**Tub**/Shower TX	*5 standby assist; supervision; stand–pivot to bathtub using transfer tub bench*
4 minimum assistance; needs cues < 25% of time for routine tasks	Problem Solving	*5 supervision; needs assistance with complex problems and occasional safety cues*
Short-term and long-term = WFL, able to recall 3/3 words; steps	Memory	*WFL*
Transfers bed to wheelchair with minimum assistance; sleep cycle = WFL	Comments	*Transfers bed to wheelchair with supervision*

Figure 3.5. Cardinal Hill Healthcare System Occupational Analysis (Adult): Case of G. C.

Client Name: _G. C._ _____ Client #: _____

Initial Comments		Discharge Comments
	Instrumental ADLs	
Drove/independent prior to CVA	Community Mobility	_Driving not recommended at this time 2° to left inattention_
Walked for exercise prior; independent prior	Health Management	_Needs supervision for medications_
Assisted with laundry and cleaning house; did all yard work	Home Management	_Able to assist with laundry; yard work not recommended at this time 2° to safety_
Performed bill paying; did most electronically; independent prior	Financial Management	_Needs assistance with money management and check-writing_
See profile; woodworking, etc.	Leisure	_Plans to resume with assistance_
Impulsive at times with transfers and dressing; able to verbally state appropriate emergency response plans	Safety	_Impulsivity remains; however, client is less impulsive and is able to slow down and assess safety of situation at times_
Assists with caring for pet (cat)	Comments	_Plans to assist with cat/resume as able_
	Movement Function	
Supervision, EOB/CGA; steadying while dressing	Sitting—Static/Dynamic	_Independent for static balance; close SBA and supervision for dynamic sitting balance_
Minimal assistance/moderate assistance	Standing—Static/Dynamic	_Supervision – CGA/minimal assistance_
Left shoulder subluxation – mild	Joint Stability and Skeletal Mobility	_No left shoulder subluxation_

Figure 3.5. Cardinal Hill Healthcare System Occupational Analysis (Adult): Case of G. C. _(continued)._

(continued)

Client Name: _G. C._ _____ Client #: _____

Initial Comments   **Discharge Comments**

Initial Comments		Discharge Comments
R = able; WFL through full ROM *L = unable 2° to ↓ distal control; trace hand grasp; also poor proximal strength; w/c level*	Place can on shelf	*R = able; WFL; w/c level* *L = unable; however, client has minimal hand grasp and ↑ proximal movement and strength*
R = able; WFL with supervision for safety 2° to balance and impulsivity *L = unable 2° to poor hand grasp strength, ↓ coordination and motor control; w/c level*	Retrieve item from floor	*R = able; WFL; client demonstrates ↑ balance and ↑ safety awareness* *L = able to pick up pair of socks with primitive grasp pattern & ↑ time (wearing seatbelt w/c level)*
R = able while stabilizing between legs *L = unable; w/c level*	Screw lid on jar	*R = able while stabilizing between legs* *LUE attempts to help stabilize jar; w/c level*
R = able/WFL L = N/T 2° to R hand dominant	Comb back of head	*R = able/WFL; L = N/T 2° to R hand dominant; w/c level*
R = able/WFL L = N/T; w/c level	Write name	*R = able/WFL L = N/T; w/c level*
R = able/WFL through full ROM with adequate strength; lifted bag from floor to top of table *L = U/A 2° to ↓ strength, motor control, grasp, and coordination*	Lift grocery bag	*R = able/WFL through full ROM with adequate strength* *L = U/A 2° to ↓ strength, motor control, grasp, and coordination*
RUE AROM = WFL; LUE PROM = WFL; LUE = active mvt. in shldr & elbow (2-/5), trace extension, trace finger flexion; LUE = non-fx'l	Comments	*LUE = shldr & elbow (3-/5), wrist extension = (2-/5), uses LUE as a stabilizer during fx'l wrist activities and automatically integrates LUE into fx'l activities at times; uses to stabilize body for balance and paper when writing or items on meal tray.*

Figure 3.5. Cardinal Hill Healthcare System Occupational Analysis (Adult): Case of G. C. *(continued).*

Client Name: _G. C._   Client #: _____

Initial Comments   **Discharge Comments**

Initial Comments		Discharge Comments
Poor; SOB with dressing, needed 2 rest breaks	Energy for Task	_Fair, for occupational participation_
Gross and fine motor: R = WFL; L = impaired, able to use as stabilizer with cues, no automatic use or fx'l grasp	Coordination	_R = WFL; L = impaired, but improving; has a minimal grasp_
L _N/T_ R _94_ _N/T_	Grip Strength/Lateral Pinch lbs/3 Jaw Chuck	L _12_ - - R _96_ - -
Impaired; environmental stimuli is distracting; uses tools appropriately, no difficulty with initiation or sequencing	Knowledge/Organization of Task	_WFL_
Impaired; has difficulty adjusting 2° to impulsivity & inattention; needs ↑ time to adapt to environmental stimuli	Adaptation/Praxis	_WFL; increased insight and ability to problem solve, motor plan, etc., in order to adapt_
Unable to accommodate at times efficiently and safely 2° to impulsivity	Comments	_Improved ability to accommodate, adjust, and benefit_
WFL; appropriate responses, good eye contact, can express complex ideas	**Social Interaction Skills**	_WFL_
	Cognitive & Affective	
Alert/distracted at times in noisy environment, requiring minimal cues	Level of Arousal/Attention	_Alert/isn't as easily distracted as on admission_
Oriented to person, place, time, & situation	Orientation	_0 x 4_
Motivated to regain independence, return home with wife, and resume occupations; impaired impulse control with transfers and during dressing tasks. Appears to have good self-esteem in resuming self-care, has difficulty controlling emotions at times (labile); expresses anxiety about having another PE or CVA.	Energy and Drive	_Excited about returning home and resuming daily activities and occupations. Improved self-concept ↓ lability. Motivated to continue with therapy on outpatient basis._

Figure 3.5. Cardinal Hill Healthcare System Occupational Analysis (Adult): Case of G. C. _(continued)._   _(continued)_

Client Name: *G. C.* Client #: _____

Initial Comments   **Discharge Comments**

Initial Comments		Discharge Comments
TBA further; able to complete money management with minimal cues; unrealistic expectations of time frame of progress; client appears to demonstrate healthy coping skills	**Higher Level Cognition**	*Needs supervision; able to perform check-writing but some difficulty with counting out change; independent with medication routine; good coping skills continue*
RUE = WFL *LUE = light touch, temp., and proprioception = impaired*	**Sensory**	*LUE = temp. & proprioception = intact* *Light touch = impaired*
Wears glasses at all times; no hemianopsia present; no changes since CVA; further visual screen not needed	**Visual**	*WFL*
Left inattention – mild; ↓ body awareness, Impaired sensory interpretation	**Perception**	*Left inattention has improved but still present*
Left shoulder pain occasionally, rates a 4/10	**Pain**	*Reports ↓ LUE pain, still rates a 4/10 but pain is less often*
Intact; Left hand edema = mild	**Skin Integrity**	*Intact; no left hand edema*
	Comments	

	Pre	Post		Pre	Post		Pre	Post		Pre	Post		Pre	Post		Pre	Post
HR	*88*	*101*	O₂	*N/T*	*93*	RPD	*N/T*	*N/T*	HR	*84*	*98*	O₂	*N/T*	*N/T*	RPD	*N/T*	*N/T*

Comments

Figure 3.5. Cardinal Hill Healthcare System Occupational Analysis (Adult): Case of G. C. *(continued).*

Client Name: _G. C._   Client #: _____

Initial Comments   **Discharge Comments**

How do the risks interfere with participation in occupation?

Client presents with decreased ability to participate in meaningful occupations such as self-care, yard work, laundry, and woodworking because of decreased balance, motor control, strength, energy, sensation, perception, pain, ROM, coordination, problem solving, and is a safety risk because of impulsivity and the aforementioned factors.

How has occupational therapy facilitated participation in occupation in client's environment?

OT has facilitated participation in occupation by providing education in BADLs and IADLs and issued AE as appropriate. OT has provided family education with client's wife and had wife demonstrate appropriate techniques in assisting client at home. OT intervention has included orthotic fabrication, neuromuscular re-education, functional electrical stimulation, and safety education with emphasis on preparation for occupational participation. Client participated in home management and leisure activities that he identified as occupations he wanted to resume.

Equipment:

TBA prior to discharge

Equipment provided:

Reacher, versa-frame commode rails, and transfer tub bench Elastic shoelaces

Goals met:

1–6, 9

Goals not met:

7, 8, 10

ELOS:

3 weeks

Number of visits:

N/A for inpatient stay

Reason for discharge:

LOS complete; goals met

D/C recommendations/referrals:

OT recommends 24-hour supervision for bathroom transfers, continued outpatient OT, and no driving at this time.

Therapist's Signature	Date	Therapist's Signature	Date

Figure 3.5. Cardinal Hill Healthcare System Occupational Analysis (Adult): Case of G. C. *(continued).*

Note. CVA = cerebral vascular accident; ADLs = activities of daily living; w/c = wheelchair; EOB = edge of bed; E/W/S = edge of bed/wheelchair/supine; UB = upper body; LB = lower body; WFL = within functional limits; CGA = contact guard assistance; SBA = standby assistance; ROM = range of motion; LUE = left upper extremity; N/T = not tested; R = right; U/A = unable; RUE = right upper extremity; AROM = active range of motion; PROM = passive range of motion; shldr = shoulder; fx'l = functional; SOB = shortness of breath; L = left; O x 4 = oriented x 4; PE = pulmonary embolism; temp. = temperature; HR = heart rate; O_2 = oxygen; RPD = rate of perceived dyspnea; OT = occupational therapy; BADLs = basic activities of daily living; IADLs = instrumental activities of daily living; AE = adaptive equipment; ELOS = estimated length of stay; LOS = length of stay; D/C = discharge.

Cardinal Hill Healthcare System
Inpatient Intervention Plan

Client: _G. C._   Client #: _____   DOB: _12-05-36_

Admit Date: _6-6-05_

Decreased satisfaction/ability to participate in the following occupations:

☑ Eating	☑ Community Mobility	☐ Shopping
☑ Grooming	☑ Safety/Emergency Response	☐ Education
☑ Bathing	☐ Financial Management	☑ Work
☑ Dressing	☑ Health Management	☑ Leisure/Play
☑ Toilet Transfer	☑ Home Management	☑ Functional Mobility
☑ Tub/Shower Transfer	☑ Social Participation	

Performance risks that interfere with participation in occupations:

☑ Problem Solving	☑ Neuromuscular/Movement	☐ Skin Integrity
☐ Memory	☐ Oral Motor/Dysphagia	☑ Pain
☑ Cognition	☑ Mobility	☑ Organization/Adaptability
☑ Posture	☑ Coordination	☑ Sensory Functions
☑ Energy/Endurance	☑ Strength/Effort	☐ Vision Functions
☑ Perception		

Strengths (contextual influences): _friendly, motivated; supportive wife_

Short-term goals: _(1 week) 1) Client will perform upper body dressing with minimal assistance, EOB, using hemi-technique. 2) Client will complete grooming with set-up/supervision, w/c level. 3) Client will don socks with set-up using crossed leg technique w/c level._

4) Client will perform leisure activity of his choice standing at table for 5 minutes with minimal assistance.

Discharge Goals/Rehab Potential: Client will demonstrate:

☑ 1. Eating with _setup_ _____ using _____

☑ 2. Grooming with _independence_ _____ using _____ ☑ w/c level ☐ walker level ☐ standing

☑ 3. Bathing with _set-up/supervision_ _____ using _long sponge if needed_ ☐ sponge bath ☑ tub bath

☑ 4. Upper body dressing with _setup_ _____ using _hemi-technique_ ☑ EOB ☐ w/c level ☐ supine

☑ 5. Lower body dressing with _setup_ _____ using _hemi-technique_ ☑ EOB ☐ w/c level ☐ supine

☑ 6. Toilet transfer with _standby assistance/supervision_ using _elevated commode rails_ ☐ w/c level ☑ walker level

☑ 7. Tub/shower transfer with _minimal assistance_ using _transfer tub bench_ ☐ w/c level ☑ walker level

☑ 8. Problem solving with _independence_

☐ 9. Memory with _____

☑ 10. Light homemaking activities with _minimal assistance_ using _adaptive equipment as needed_ ☑ w/c level ☐ walker level

Client/Family will:

☑ 11. Demonstrate knowledge to assist client with ADLs as needed

☑ 12. Perform home program with _independence_ assistance

☑ 13. Participate in community outing with _supervision_ assistance ☑ w/c level ☑ walker level – _to be assessed_

☑ 14. Demonstrate use of equipment with _minimal, as needed_ assistance

☑ 15. Engage in leisure exploration and/or participation with _supervision/standby assistance; including woodworking_

☑ 16. _Use LUE as a stabilizer during functional activities 50% of the time._

☑ 17. _Fold laundry wheelchair level with setup and supervision._

Figure 3.6. Cardinal Hill Healthcare System Inpatient Intervention Plan: Case of G. C.

Plan of Treatment/Education in:

☑ ADL	☑ Work/Productive Activities	☑ Psychosocial	☑ Positioning
☑ Neuromuscular Movement	☑ Cognitive Activities	☑ Sensory Activities	☐ Aquatics
☑ Skin/Edema	☑ Splinting/Casting	☑ Perceptual Tasks	☑ Leisure
☑ Modalities	☐ Oral Motor/Swallowing	☐ Re-Evaluation	☐ Co-Treat
☑ Adaptive Equipment	☑ D/C Planning	☐ Home Visit	☐ Other
☑ Home Program	☑ Client/Caregiver Education	☑ Home Safety/Equipment	

Frequency: _BID-TID 5–6 days per week_   Duration: _3 weeks_

Medical Diagnosis: _CVA with left hemiplegia_

OT Diagnosis: _↓ occupational participation, ↓ independence with BADLs and IADLs_

Contraindications/Precautions: _cardiac, fall_

I certify that occupational therapy services are necessary under a plan to be periodically reviewed by me and while the patient is under my care.

_____	_____	_____	_____
Date	Therapist's Signature	Accepted Date	Physician's Signature

Figure 3.6. Cardinal Hill Healthcare System Inpatient Intervention Plan: Case of G. C. *(continued).*

Note. EOB = edge of bed; w/c = wheelchair; ADL = activities of daily living; LUE = left upper extremity; D/C = discharge; BID-TID = 2 times per day/3 times per day; CVA = cerebral vascular accident; OT = occupational therapy; BADLs = basic activities of daily living; IADLs = instrumental activities of daily living.

Cardinal Hill Healthcare System
Occupational Profile (Adult)

Client Name: *K. H.* _____ Client #: _____ DOB: *3/17/77* _____

Initial Date: *3/3/05* _____ Discharge Date: *4/7/05* _____

Diagnosis: *Closed Head Injury* _____

Precautions: *Dysphagia* _____

1. Client lives ☑ with ☐ alone *parents* _____ in a ☑ house ☐ trailer ☐ apt. with __*2*__ steps to enter ☐ R/ ☐ L handrail; __*2*__ stories; _____ steps inside home. _____

2. Client's discharge environment, resources, and available adaptive equipment: *all equipment needed was secured during acute care* *admission. He has two children that live with him and his bedroom is on the second floor.*

3. Prior to this hospitalization, the client was ☑ I ☐ min ☐ mod in BADLs and ☑ I ☐ min ☐ mod in IADLs. Client needed assistance with *no occupations.*

4. A typical day consists of: wake up time *8–8:30* ☑ a.m. ☐ p.m.; ☐ volunteer ☐ work; bedtime *11:30* ☐ a.m. ☑ p.m.
   In the am. wake up, eat, shower every other day, groom, dress. Get the kids ready, go to work. Help make dinner. Go out with friends.
   On the weekend, he tends to wake around 9:00 am, get his kids breakfast, cuts the grass, does household chores, grocery shops, rides ATV,
   fishes and sees friends.

5. What activities do you participate in for fun and how often? *Shopping, occasional TV, watch kids play, fishing, baseball, volleyball,* *ATV riding.*

6. How do you learn best? (In rehab you will be learning new things. Do you learn best by reading, watching a video?) _____
   "demonstration first and then practice"

7. How familiar are you with technology? *I use the computer for e-mail and Web searching.* _____

8. What motivates you to improve? *I want to raise my girls and see them grow up.* _____

9. How are you coping with your current status? *I think I am doing okay.* _____

Initial Comments   **Discharge Comments**

List 5 occupations you want/need to resume	Satisfaction in resuming your roles
Take care of my children	*8/10 I need help getting the kids ready*
Client's mother would like client to initiate his own routine	*8/10 Pretty good*
To be able to move around the house independently	*9/10 I can get around*
Get left arm to work as good as it can	*8/10 It can be better*
(Info obtained with assist from family secondary to client's decreased cognitive status)	

_____ _____   _____ _____
Therapist's Signature   Date   Therapist's Signature   Date

Figure 3.7. Cardinal Hill Healthcare System Occupational Profile (Adult): Case of K. H.
Note. ATV = all-terrain vehicle; R/L = right/left; I = independent; min = minimum; mod = moderate; BADLs = basic activities of daily living; IADLs = instrumental activities of daily living.

Cardinal Hill Healthcare System
Occupational Analysis (Adult)

Client Name: _K. H._ Client #: _____ DOB: _3/17/77_

Initial Date: _3/3/05_ Discharge Date: _4/7/05_

Diagnosis: _Closed Head Injury_

Precautions: _Dysphagia_

Occupational Analysis:

Initial Comments		**Discharge Comments**
	Basic ADLs	
5 – setup to cut tough foods	Eating	5 – setup for bite size secondary to dysphagia
5 – verbal cues for task initiation, setup	Grooming	Independent, able to initiate appropriately
5 – verbal cues to sequence steps of task	Bathing	Standby assist for safety in shower, able to shave in shower
5 – setup to orient clothes and sequence steps of task	**E**/W/S Dressing UB **E**/W/S	Supervision for clothes selection and sequencing of dressing
5 – takes extra time and cues to stay on task	**E**/W/S Dressing LB **E**/W/S	Independent, including shoe tying
5 – secondary to decreased balance	Toilet TX	Independent with commode transfer
5 – requires supervision for decreased balance	**Tub**/Shower TX	Standby assist for safety
4 – min assist for timely decisions and initiation of tasks	Problem Solving	Client able to follow 3-step directions and solve simple BADL problems
Severely delayed short- & long-term memory to recognize staff and follow daily schedule	Memory	Severe delay in STM and LTM interfering with new learning and safety
Deficits in sleep/rest cycle and transfers	Comments	Sleep cycle only slightly delayed now

Figure 3.8. Cardinal Hill Healthcare System Occupational Analysis (Adult): Case of K. H.

(continued)

Client Name: _K. H._   Client #: _____

Initial Comments   **Discharge Comments**

Initial Comments	Instrumental ADLs	Discharge Comments
Dependent for driving	Community Mobility	_Recommend client does not drive until driving evaluation is completed_
Minimal assist and verbal cues to follow home exercise program	Health Management	_Setup assist for medication management, verbal cues for home program performance_
Moderate assist for light cleaning: dusting, washing dishes, max assist for shopping and cooking	Home Management	_Increases noted as client can now perform laundry, set table, dust, and perform light cleaning_
Moderate assist for counting less than $20 due to vision deficits	Financial Management	_Dependent for money management. Client able to purchase items with minimal change needed/given_
Verbal cues to initiate leisure participation	Leisure	_Increased leisure pursuits including shopping and going out with friends_
Moderate delays in safety awareness and proper response to unsafe situation	Safety	_24-hr supervision recommend secondary to memory and awareness_
Requires supervision for all IADLs	Comments	
	Movement Function	
WFL for sitting both static and dynamic	Sitting—Static/Dynamic	_WFL for both_
Standby assist for standing especially with grooming at sink	Standing—Static/Dynamic	_Supervision required for both secondary to decreased balance and safety judgment_
Half-finger subluxation at left shoulder	Joint Stability and Skeletal Mobility	_Subluxation is resolved_

Figure 3.8. Cardinal Hill Healthcare System Occupational Analysis (Adult): Case of K. H. _(continued)._

Client Name: _K. H._ _____ Client #: _____

Initial Comments   **Discharge Comments**

Initial Comments	Task	Discharge Comments
LUE – not functional, RUE – WFL	Place can on shelf	_Independent bilaterally at shoulder height from standing_
LUE – not functional, RUE – WFL	Retrieve item from floor	_Independent bilaterally from stance_
LUE – not functional, right RUE – WFL	Screw lid on jar	_Independent with BUE_
LUE – not functional, RUE – WFL	Comb back of head	_Independent with BUE_
Client wrote name with RUE	Write name	_Client demonstrated increased control with signature_
LUE – unable secondary to decreased muscle function, RUE – WFL _Bag lifted from floor to counter height_	Lift grocery bag	_WNL for RUE, unable with LUE secondary to decreased strength_ _Bag lifted from floor to counter height_
RUE – AROM WFL, LUE – shoulder flex 45° _Compensatory movement patterns noted_ _Abd. 45° Elev. 5°_ _Elbow flexion 63°_ _Digit flex/ext, oppos – WNL_ _Pron./Sup. – WFL_	Comments	_RUE – WFL, LUE shoulder flex – 90°_ _Compensatory movement patterns noted_ _Abd. 80°_ _Elbow flex/ext – WNL_ _Pron./Sup. ext – WFL_ _Digit flex, ext – WFL_

Figure 3.8. Cardinal Hill Healthcare System Occupational Analysis (Adult): Case of K. H. *(continued)*.

(continued)

Client Name: _K. H._ _____ Client #: _____

Initial Comments   **Discharge Comments**

Initial Comments								Measure	Discharge Comments							
WFL for ADLs and leisure participation								Energy for Task	*WFL, decreased attention with increased activity noted*							
LUE – limited secondary to decreased ROM, RUE – WFL								Coordination	*Increased coordination for writing and ADLs, 9-hole peg test 69.8 seconds LUE*							
L	*18*			R	*50*			Grip Strength/Lateral Pinch lbs/3 Jaw Chuck	L	*32#*	*10#*	*8#*	R	*55#*	*17#*	*23#*
Poor to choose ADL item and heed task, poor initiation and continuing								Knowledge/Organization of Task	*Slight deficit now in ability to initiate ADLs*							
Moderate deficit to adjust/adapt/benefit								Adaptation/Praxis	*Intact in ability to adjust/adapt and benefit to BADLs*							
Client relies on verbal cues to complete ADLs therefore unable to assess praxis skills								Comments	*Client able to complete BADLs without cues, requires min assist for IADLs*							
Client able to express basic wants and needs, maintains eye contact and appropriate facial responses								**Social Interaction Skills**	*Social skills remain slightly impaired but increases noted in ability to discuss basic concepts with peers, combative behavior noted x 1*							
								Cognitive & Affective								
Arousal slightly decreased affecting follow-through during ADLs								Level of Arousal/Attention	*Slight decrease in attention with increased time to complete task needed*							
Oriented to person and place								Orientation	*Oriented x 4*							
Poor for motivation to complete ADLs, fair motivation for therapy participation								Energy and Drive	*Requires maximum encouragement to participate in therapy*							

Figure 3.8. Cardinal Hill Healthcare System Occupational Analysis (Adult): Case of K. H. *(continued).*

Client Name: *K. H.* _____ Client #: _____

Initial Comments   **Discharge Comments**

Initial Comments		Discharge Comments
Client requires verbal cues for basic tasks	**Higher Level Cognition**	*Moderate deficit to complete nonroutine tasks and learn new skills*
Client reports LUE feels same as RUE, decreased local response to light touch, deep pressure and temperature	**Sensory**	*Intact to light touch, deep pressure and temperature in LUE, RUE remains intact*
Reports double vision, appt. with neuro-ophthalmologist 3/10/05, required verbal cues secondary to depth perception deficits	**Visual**	*Continues to complain of double vision. Depth perception slightly impaired for grooming*
Figure ground deficits with grooming noted for deodorant application	**Perception**	*Decreased visual attention to peripheral field and left neglect noted at times*
LUE shoulder pain with movement 5/10	**Pain**	*No c/o pain*
WNL	**Skin Integrity**	*Intact*
Client displays decreased body image during movement tasks	Comments	*Body image and self-concept intact*

	Pre	Post		Pre	Post		Pre	Post		Pre	Post		Pre	Post		Pre	Post
HR	82	89	O₂	90	90	RPD	2	2	HR	85	86	O₂	93	94	RPD	1	1

Sats measured before and after a.m. ADLs	Comments	*Sats measured before and after a.m. ADLs*

Figure 3.8. Cardinal Hill Healthcare System Occupational Analysis (Adult): Case of K. H. *(continued).*

(continued)

Client Name: _K. H._ _____ Client #: _____

Initial Comments	**Discharge Comments**
How do the risks interfere with participation in occupation?	How has occupational therapy facilitated participation in occupation in client's environment?
Decreased ability to perform BADLs and IADLs secondary to decreased memory, energy for task and LUE function.	*Client can now return to home environment and participate in valued occupations with 24-hr supervision as increases are noted in LUE function, strength, ROM, and coordination. Increased initiation to complete BADLs and IADLs noted. Family demonstrates competency in supervising completion of home program and supervision requirements.*

Equipment:
none at this time

Equipment provided:
home program

Goals met:

STGs # 1,2,3,4,5, and added 1,2,3; LTGs 2,3,5

Goals not met:

LTGs 1,4

ELOS:
4 weeks

Number of visits:

N/A for inpatient admission

Reason for discharge:
met maximum potential for inpatient rehabilitation at this time

D/C recommendations/referrals:
outpatient occupational therapy, driving evaluation recommended

_____   _____   _____   _____
Therapist's Signature   Date   Therapist's Signature   Date

Figure 3.8. Cardinal Hill Healthcare System Occupational Analysis (Adult): Case of K. H. *(continued).*

Note. ADLs = activities of daily living; min = minimum; BADLs = basic activities of daily living; E/W/S = edge of bed/wheelchair/supine; STM = short-term memory; LTM = long-term memory; max = maximum; IADLs = instrumental activities of daily living; WFL = within functional limits; LUE = left upper extremity; RUE = right upper extremity; BUE = both upper extremities; oppos = opposite; WNL = within normal limits; AROM = active range of motion; Abd = abduction; flex = flexion; Elev. = elevation; ext = extension; Pron./Sup. = pronation/supination; L = left; R = right; c/o = complaints of; HR = heart rate; O_2 = oxygen; RPD = rate of perceived dyspnea; Sats = oxygen saturation; ROM = range of motion; STG = short-term goal; LTG = long-term goal; ELOS = estimated length of stay; D/C = discharge.

Cardinal Hill Healthcare System
Inpatient Intervention Plan

Client: _K. H._   Client #: _____   DOB: _3/17/77_

Admit Date: _3/3/05_

Decreased satisfaction/ability to participate in the following occupations:

☑ Eating	☑ Community Mobility	☑ Shopping
☑ Grooming	☑ Safety/Emergency Response	☐ Education
☑ Bathing	☑ Financial Management	☑ Work
☑ Dressing	☑ Health Management	☑ Leisure/Play
☑ Toilet Transfer	☑ Home Management	☑ Functional Mobility
☑ Tub/Shower Transfer	☑ Social Participation	

Performance risks that interfere with participation in occupations:

☑ Problem Solving	☑ Neuromuscular/Movement	☐ Skin Integrity
☑ Memory	☑ Oral Motor/Dysphagia	☑ Pain
☑ Cognition	☑ Mobility	☑ Organization/Adaptability
☐ Posture	☑ Coordination	☑ Sensory Functions
☑ Energy/Endurance	☑ Strength/Effort	☑ Vision Functions
☑ Perception		

Strengths (contextual influences): _decreased energy to initiate BADLs, has desire to return to familiar role._

Short-term goals: _1. Client will be able to transfer to toilet with modified independence, and perform toilet hygiene while using commode bars demonstrating improved balance. 2. Client will be able to lay out clothes and grooming items independently to sequence steps of dressing. 3. Client will demonstrate ability to follow adapted dressing techniques to independently dress self and mod assist with fasteners._

Discharge Goals/Rehab Potential: Client will demonstrate:

☑ 1. Eating with _independently_ using _____
☑ 2. Grooming with _supervision for shaving_ using _____ ☐ w/c level ☐ walker level ☑ standing
☑ 3. Bathing with _standby assist_ using _____ ☐ sponge bath ☑ tub bath
☑ 4. Upper body dressing with _independently_ using _____ ☑ EOB ☐ w/c level ☐ supine
☑ 5. Lower body dressing with _independently_ using _____ ☑ EOB ☐ w/c level ☐ supine
☑ 6. Toilet transfer with _independently in standing_ using _____ ☐ w/c level ☐ walker level
☑ 7. Tub/shower transfer with _independently in standing_ using _____ ☐ w/c level ☐ walker level
☑ 8. Problem solving with _minimum assist to complete IADLs._
☑ 9. Memory with _minimum assist to follow simple nonhabitual commands to complete IADLs._
☑ 10. Light homemaking activities with _independently complete_ using _____ ☐ w/c level ☐ walker level
simple meal prep and cleaning with supervision while ambulating.

Client/Family will:
☑ 11. Demonstrate knowledge to assist client with ADLs as needed
☑ 12. Perform home program with _minimum_ assistance _to cue for daily completion_
☑ 13. Participate in community outing with _supervision_ assistance ☑ w/c level ☑ walker level
☐ 14. Demonstrate use of equipment with _____ assistance
☑ 15. Engage in leisure exploration and/or participation with _supervision for safety_
☑ 16. _Client will be able to dress children and prepare a simple breakfast for them with supervision._
☐ 17. _____

Figure 3.9. Cardinal Hill Healthcare System Inpatient Intervention Plan: Case of K. H.

(continued)

Plan of Treatment/Education in:

☑ ADL	☑ Work/Productive Activities	☑ Psychosocial	☐ Positioning
☑ Neuromuscular Movement	☑ Cognitive Activities	☑ Sensory Activities	☐ Aquatics
☐ Skin/Edema	☐ Splinting/Casting	☑ Perceptual Tasks	☑ Leisure
☐ Modalities	☑ Oral Motor/Swallowing	☑ Re-Evaluation	☑ Co-Treat
☑ Adaptive Equipment	☑ D/C Planning	☑ Home Visit	☐ Other
☑ Home Program	☑ Client/Caregiver Education	☑ Home Safety/Equipment	

Frequency: *2x daily 6 days a week*   Duration: *4 weeks*

Medical Diagnosis: *CHI*

OT Diagnosis: *Decreased ability to participate in BADLs and IADLs, especially care of children.*

Contraindications/Precautions: *dysphagia, LUE subluxation*

I certify that occupational therapy services are necessary under a plan to be periodically reviewed by me and while the patient is under my care.

Date	Therapist's Signature	Accepted Date	Physician's Signature

Figure 3.9. Cardinal Hill Healthcare System Inpatient Intervention Plan: Case of K. H. *(continued).*

Note. BADLs = basic activities of daily living; mod = moderate; assist. = assistance; w/c = wheelchair; EOB = edge of bed; IADLs = instrumental activities of daily living; DC = discharge; CHI = closed head injury; OT = occupational therapist; LUE = left upper extremity.

Cardinal Hill Healthcare System
Occupational Profile (Pediatric)

Client Name: _C. C._   Client #: _____   DOB: _10/01/91_

Initial Date: _06/18/04_   Discharge Date: _11/20/04_

Diagnosis: _Dyspraxia, fine motor and handwriting difficulties_

Precautions: _None noted_

Occupational Profile:

1. Client lives with _his mother and two older sisters_ in a ☑ house ☐ trailer ☐ apt. with _____ steps to enter
   ☐ R/ ☐ L handrail; _____ stories; _____ steps inside home. _____

2. A typical day consists of: wake up time _7:00_ ☑ a.m. ☐ p.m.; bedtime _10:00_ ☐ a.m. ☑ p.m.
   Go to school (in the fall), baseball practice, socialize with friends, chores, homework (when school is in session).

3. What activities do you participate in for fun and how often? _Play sports, play video games_

4. How do you learn best? (In rehab you will be learning new things. Do you learn best by reading, watching a video?) _____
   Demonstration

5. How familiar are you with technology? _Use the computer every day._

6. What motivates you to improve? _I don't know._

7. How are you and your family coping with your current status? _I just don't want people to think I'm stupid._

Initial Comments   **Discharge Comments**

List 5 occupations you want/need to resume	Satisfaction in resuming your roles
Write neater	8/10 It's better than it was
Make own snack/meals	9/10 I can make a lot of different things now
Improve posture	8/10 I still have to be reminded now and then
Tie shoes tighter/button buttons	10/10 It's easy
Make my hands stronger	9/10 This is a lot better

| Therapist's Signature | Date | Therapist's Signature | Date |

Figure 3.10. Cardinal Hill Healthcare System Occupational Profile (Pediatric): Case of C. C.

Cardinal Hill Healthcare System
Occupational Analysis (Pediatric)

Client Name: _C. C._   Client #: _____   DOB: _____

Initial Date: _____   Discharge Date: _____

Diagnosis: _Dyspraxia, fine motor problems_   Precautions: _None noted_ _____

Age: _12_   Grade in School: _7_   Physician: _____

Occupational Analysis:

Initial Comments   **Discharge Comments**

Initial Comments	Basic ADLs	Discharge Comments
Child evaluated for 60 minutes and accompanied by his mother who acted as primary informant for this evaluation. His mother is concerned with his handwriting and "processing" abilities.		*Parent and child satisfied with child's improvement.*
ADLs: Activities that are oriented toward taking care of one's own body (adapted from Rogers & Holm, 1994)	**Basic ADLs**	*NA*
Child independent with feeding, but has difficulty using utensils (e.g., spreading with knife)	Eating/Oral Motor	*Child independent, safe & neat with knife, fork, & spoon*
Child is independent and age appropriate	Grooming	*Same as initial evaluation*
Child is independent and age appropriate	Bathing/Transfer	*Same as initial evaluation*
Child requires moderate assistance with buttons	Dressing Upper Body	*Child independent with dress shirt buttons*
Child requires minimum assistance to tie shoes tightly	Dressing Lower Body	*Child independent with shoe tying. Shoes staying tied.*
Child is independent and age appropriate	Toilet Training/Transfer	*Same as initial evaluation*
Child has difficulty organizing ADL tasks in a.m.	Problem Solving/Memory	*Child utilizing schedule with minimal adult verbal cues*
Child late for school or forgets school materials at home. Child unable to make own snack/ simple meal.	Comments	*Morning routine schedule used to assist child with a.m. ADLs, chores, & organizing school supplies*

Age Equivalent	Percentile	Standard Score	ADL Test	Age Equivalent	Percentile	Standard Score
NA	*NA*	*NA*	*NA*	*NA*	*NA*	*NA*

Figure 3.11. Cardinal Hill Healthcare System Occupational Analysis (Pediatric): Case of C. C.

(continued)

Client Name: _C. C._ _____ Client #: _____

Initial Comments   **Discharge Comments**

Initial Comments	Instrumental ADLs	Discharge Comments
Child is age appropriate.	Community Mobility	*Same as initial evaluation*
Child requires frequent reminders to complete chores.	Home Management	*Child utilizing chore schedule with parent assistance*
Child chooses age-appropriate options (e.g., sports).	Play Exploration	*Same as initial evaluation*
Child plays independently and with peers.	Play Participation	*Same as initial evaluation*
Child is described as cautious during play.	Safety	*Same as initial evaluation*
NA	Comments	*NA*
	Movement Function	
Inadequate: maintains for 10 seconds	Supine Flexion Posture	*Adequate: Child maintains posture for 30 seconds.*
Inadequate: Unable to obtain	Prone Extension Posture	*Progressed: Child maintains posture for 20 seconds.*
Sits in chair independently with arms propped on table and posterior pelvic tilt	Sitting Posture/Balance	*Upright posture with use of wedge on chair*
Able to obtain & maintain age-appropriate positions	Developmental Positions	*Same as initial evaluation*
Upper-body muscle tone & strength: functional	Muscle Functions	*Same as initial evaluation*

Figure 3.11. Cardinal Hill Healthcare System Occupational Analysis (Pediatric): Case of C. C. *(continued).*

(continued)

Client Name: _C. C._   Client #: _____

Initial Comments   **Discharge Comments**

Initial Comments	Movement Function	Discharge Comments
Upper-body active range of motion: normal	**Movement Function**	*Same as initial evaluation*
Age appropriate	Reflexes	*Same as initial evaluation*
Scapular instability (winging, noted during writing)	Comments	*Activation of scapular muscles for joint stability when reminded*
Appropriate	Energy for Task	*Same as initial evaluation*
Adequate	Coordination	*Same as initial evaluation*
Difficulty with buttons. Child is slow to complete manipulation tasks.	Manipulation	*Independent with buttons. Child demonstrates slow/deliberate completion of manipulation tasks.*
Inadequate: Letters formed from bottom to top. Alignment is poor. Spacing is close together.	Visual Motor	*Child continues to form letters from bottom to top. Alignment & spacing are now adequate.*
Inadequate: Difficulty imitating novel motor tasks.	Adaptation/Praxis	*Continues to have difficulty with novel motor activities.*
Right hand dominates, uses immature quadripod grasp.	Comments	*Progressed: Child uses pencil grip to support pencil grasp.*

Age Equivalent	Percentile	Standard Score	Motor Test	Age Equivalent	Percentile	Standard Score
10 year 2 months	*NA*	*9*		*11 years 2 months*	*NA*	*12*
Age Equivalent	Percentile	Standard Score	Motor Test	Age Equivalent	Percentile	Standard Score
8 years 10 months	*25*	*90*		*11 years*	*53*	*101*

Figure 3.11. Cardinal Hill Healthcare System Occupational Analysis (Pediatric): Case of C. C. *(continued).*

Client Name: _C. C._   Client #: _____

Initial Comments   **Discharge Comments**

Initial Comments		Discharge Comments
Child readily greets therapist. Eye contact: good	**Social Interaction Skills**	Same as initial evaluation
Child presents with decreased arousal level	**Cognitive Perceptual & Affective**	Child continues to present with decreased arousal level
Child maintains attention for evaluation	Level of Arousal/Attention	Child able to maintain attention for post-test
Participates in testing tasks. Good impulse control.	Energy & Drive	Same as initial evaluation
Parent reports child is easily distracted at home and school.	Comments	Parent reports increased attention for homework and chores.

			Sensory			
Ability to perceive sensory input. When children receive inaccurate or unreliable sensory input, their ability to process the information and create appropriate responses is disrupted. *(Adapted from Dunn et al., 1999)*			**Sensory**	NA		

Typical	Atypical		Sensory Test	Typical	Atypical	
Movement sensitivity Seeks sensation Visual sensitivity	Auditory filtering Low energy/weak			Movement sensitivity Seeks sensation, Visual sensitivity, Low energy/weak	Auditory filtering	

Child demonstrates frequent postural shifts when sitting, parent reports child often "fidgets," child easily distracted by noise.	Comments	Progressed with the use of wedge in chair & scheduled "motor breaks" to allow child to get up and move periodically.

			Perception			
			Perception			

Age Equivalent	Percentile	Standard Score	Perception Test	Age Equivalent	Percentile	Standard Score

Child able to maintain fixation on moving target. Frequent overshooting noted with visual saccades.	**Visual**	Progressed with speed of reading & ability to read one page without losing place.
Child does not wear glasses. Child had visual exam 6 months ago. Child demonstrates frequent squinting during visual motor tasks.	Comments	Child continues to squint. Referral made to optometrist.

Figure 3.11. Cardinal Hill Healthcare System Occupational Analysis (Pediatric): Case of C. C. *(continued).*

(continued)

Client Name: *C. C.* _____ Client #: _____

Initial Comments   **Discharge Comments**

How do the risks interfere with participation in occupation?

Child presents with decreased ability to perform handwriting tasks and activities of daily living secondary to difficulties with motor function, organization, and sensory processing.

How has occupational therapy facilitated participation in occupation in client's environment?

Child demonstrates improvements with visual motor skills for handwriting and ability to complete activities of daily living with increased independence. Family demonstrates ability to support child's ability to organize activities of daily living and motor function home program.

Equipment:

None

Duration: *6 months* _____

Equipment provided:

pencil grip, wedge for chair

Number of visits: *18* _____

Reason for discharge: *Child has met all rehabilitation goals*

Discharge goals met: *All long-term goals met*

Discharge goals not met: *None*

Patient/family education: *hand strength exercises, upper-body strength exercises, education on use of pencil grip & chair wedge, visual motor activities, education on use of ADL schedule.*

Discharge recommendations/referrals: *Recommend continuation of use of ADL schedule. Referral to optometrist.*

_____   _____
Therapist's Signature   Date

_____   _____
Therapist's Signature   Date

Figure 3.11. Cardinal Hill Healthcare System Occupational Analysis (Pediatric): Case of C. C. *(continued).*
Note. ADLs = activities of daily living; IADLs = instrumental activities of daily living.

Cardinal Hill Healthcare System
Outpatient Intervention Plan

Client: _C. C._   Client #: _____   DOB: _10/01/91_

Decreased satisfaction/ability to participate in the following occupations:

☐ Eating	☐ Community Mobility	☑ Shopping
☐ Grooming	☐ Safety/Emergency Response	☑ Education
☐ Bathing	☐ Financial Management	☐ Work
☑ Dressing	☐ Health Management	☐ Leisure/Play
☐ Toilet Transfer	☐ Home Management	☐ Functional Mobility
☐ Tub/Shower Transfer	☐ Social Participation	

Performance risks that interfere with participation in occupations:

☐ Problem Solving	☐ Neuromuscular/Movement	☐ Skin Integrity
☐ Memory	☐ Oral Motor/Dysphagia	☐ Pain
☐ Cognition	☐ Mobility	☑ Organization/Adaptability
☑ Posture	☑ Coordination	☑ Sensory Functions
☑ Energy/Endurance	☑ Strength/Effort	☑ Vision Functions
☐ Perception		

Strengths (contextual influences): _____

Short-term goals: _1. With improved motor function, C. C. will unbutton/button ⅛" buttons on a button-down shirt he is wearing with min. assist. 75% of attempts. 2. To improve hand strength needed for ADL completion, C. C. will complete 15 minutes of graded hand strength exercises, with one rest break, each session. 3. To improve postural stabilization needed for written communication, C. C. will complete 15 minutes of exercises/activities to increase trunk strength, with one rest break, each session._

Discharge goals/rehab potential: _1. By improving motor function, C. C. will manipulate all clothing fasteners independently 75% of the time. 2. With improved visual motor skills, C.C. will independently print a legible one-paragraph letter. 3. C. C. will improve movement function to demonstrate efficient postural stabilization for sitting posture and pencil grasp when writing 75% of the time. 4. C. C. will improve knowledge and organization for IADLs to complete a simple cooking task independently and safely 75% of the time. 5. To improve therapeutic carryover in the home environment, C.C. and family will be independent with home program._

Plan of Treatment/Education in:

☑ ADL	☐ Work/Productive Activities	☐ Psychosocial Skills	☐ Positioning
☑ Neuromuscular	☐ Cognitive Activities	☐ Sensory Activities	☐ Aquatics
☐ Skin/Edema	☐ Splinting/Casting	☐ Perceptual Tasks	☐ Leisure
☐ Modalities	☐ Oral Motor/Swallowing	☑ Re-Evaluation	☐ Co-Treat
☐ Adaptive Equipment	☑ D/C Planning	☐ Home Visit	☐ HPOT
☑ Home Program	☑ Client/Caregiver Education	☐ Home Safety/Equipment	☐ Other

Figure 3.12. Cardinal Hill Healthcare System Outpatient Intervention Plan: Case of C. C.   *(continued)*

Frequency: _1x per week_   Duration: _6 months_

Medical Diagnosis: _Dyspraxia, fine motor and handwriting difficulties_

OT Diagnosis: _Decreased participation in BADLs/ADLs due to risks in motor function and adaptability_

Contraindications/Precautions: _None Noted_

I certify that occupational therapy services are necessary under a plan to be periodically reviewed by me and while the patient is under my care.

Date	Occupational Therapist's Signature	Accepted Date
	Reviewing Physician's Signature	Reviewing Physician's Signature
	Reviewing Physician's Name	Referring Physician's Name

Figure 3.12. Cardinal Hill Healthcare System Outpatient Intervention Plan: Case of C. C. *(continued).*

Note. Prep = preparation; min. = minimal; assist. = assistance; ADLs = activities of daily living; IADLs = instrumental activities of daily living; D/C = discharge; OT = occupational therapist; BADLs = basic activities of daily living; HPOT = hippotherapy.

Implementing the Cardinal Hill Occupational Participation Process: Changes in Practice

In June 2003, the new evaluation was piloted on the inpatient spinal cord unit. This helped the committee identify the need for further changes as problems surfaced through practical everyday use. The committee conducted two mandatory in-services to provide education to occupational therapy staff on the *Occupational Therapy Practice Framework: Domain and Process* (American Occupational Therapy Association, 2002; see Appendix K) and use of the new facility evaluation. Also, the committee wanted feedback from all occupational therapy staff regarding any changes needed or problems identified on the evaluation. Initial feedback from individuals not on the committee was limited. During this time, the pediatric version was modified to appropriately fit its context and apply to children.

In October 2003, all occupational therapy staff were required to use the new occupational therapy evaluation with clients. The evaluation forms and protocols were phased in over 2 months on a temporary status until December, when they became permanent. During this time, the occupational therapy staff were encouraged to provide feedback to representative committee members. The committee continually revised the evaluation, as appropriate, to make it more user friendly and comprehensive.

Challenges With Implementation

The committee had to assist the occupational therapy staff in transitioning from a medical model to a client-centered and occupation-based approach. Compromises had to be made. For example, for occupational therapists who had a difficult time accepting the new movement function grid, separate addenda to assess range of motion, strength, and sensation were created (see Appendix J). Dynamometer and pinch meter assessments were included on the occupational analysis to satisfy some occupational therapists because of the types of clients seen and the data needed for accurate measurement. Furthermore, the committee received complaints on the limited space available for the occupational therapists to write observations. The committee was able to compromise by restructuring some areas and condensing some sections. Providing the occupational therapy staff with more space for comments was the most important change made. It helped all occupational therapists accept and use the evaluation.

Another challenge evident in implementing the evaluation was simply getting all occupational therapy staff to read and refer to the *Framework* and protocols to ensure the correct and thorough evaluation of each client for improved interrater reliability. Some of the occupational therapy staff had not read the protocols, and this hindered their use of correct terminology and their understanding of the purpose of the *Framework.* Committee members developed a more-condensed version of the protocol as a solution to this problem. Committee members were available throughout the hospital to answer questions from occupational therapists struggling with the use of the evaluation.

Changes After Implementation

The following are some quotes from occupational therapists at Cardinal Hill Rehabilitation Hospital who were asked how the use of the new evaluation has changed their practice:

- I think it's more client centered and client guided than before.

- It's much more functional in treatment. I never am in the therapy room anymore; I'm either in the recreation room doing leisure or in the kitchen doing home management tasks.

- My practice has changed significantly toward a more occupation-based and client-driven focused one. I am more able to see the clients' abilities and maximize [these abilities] to help them achieve their personal goals.

- If you use the profile, the treatment plan writes itself, and it guarantees a client-centered approach. Using this evaluation, a partnership is created with the client, and I no longer impose my goals on them. This evaluation relates only to occupation and all that interferes with participation in an occupation. It clearly defines our role in the team. It has made me a better therapist.

- I believe that the new evaluation, especially the profile, allows me to build rapport with my clients more quickly. I can find out what goals are most important to the client and maximize the intervention process.

The occupational therapy practice coordinator for Cardinal Hill Healthcare System continually audits charts to determine quality and accuracy of documentation. In-services and discussions follow audits to disseminate information to improve documentation.

Evaluating the Shift to the Cardinal Hill Occupational Participation Process

Staff Insights

Eight months after the evaluation was implemented, two of the committee members—Chasity Paris, MS, OTR/L, and Dana Collins Boyle, OTR/L—conducted a survey to gain insight into the occupational therapy staff's perceptions regarding the new evaluation format. A survey method was chosen, as it provides more detailed information about the occupational therapist's perceptions on the use of the Cardinal Hill occupational participation process. The survey was distributed to all occupational therapists at Cardinal Hill Rehabilitation Hospital, excluding the researchers, to prevent bias. The staff consists of people from ages 24 to 54 years, all White. All therapists either have a bachelor's or master's degree in occupational therapy and years of practice range from 1 to 30. Fifty percent of the 40 staff members responded. All 20 surveys were included in the analysis. The survey consisted of four open-ended questions developed by the two researchers (Paris & Collins Boyle, 2005).

Mixed methods were used to analyze the data to calculate percentages and identify emerging themes. First, questionnaire results were analyzed, labeled, and cross-referenced to develop categories. Categories were processed further, with additional information and examples added to each category until the categories reached a point of saturation. During this process, the constant-comparative method was used. This method consists of constantly comparing labeled information to previous information to ensure that each piece of information is similar to all other information within the category. This process generated ideas, themes, and generalizations about each category (Bailey, 1997). Each of the four questions was analyzed individually. For each open-ended question, only responses given by four or more of the survey participants (20%) were included in the analysis. Results from the analysis are presented in Table 5.1.

Overall, the major problems and challenges identified with the evaluation implementation included learning new terminology, vagueness and subjectivity of the evaluation, lengthiness of the evaluation, and decreased respect from others (i.e., professions and insur-

Table 5.1. Occupational Therapists' Responses to the New Evaluation

Survey Question	Major Theme Identified	% Respondents Identifying Theme ($N = 20$)
1. What were the problems/challenges you encountered in implementing the new evaluation with your clients?	• Terminology of the *Framework* and new evaluation were difficult to learn or understand.	55
	• Evaluation is too subjective to display client progress or to document effectively.	40
	• Evaluation is too vague and unclear.	40
	• Evaluation is too long and takes too much time to complete.	25
	• Evaluation decreases the occupational therapist's respect from other professions, including insurance companies.	20
2. What are the positive aspects of the new evaluation?	• Evaluation is more client centered regarding treatment and goal-setting.	40
	• Evaluation is focused on occupation-based aspects of practice.	35
	• The Occupational Profile portion of the evaluation is enjoyable to use.	25
3. What helped you accept and/or embrace the new evaluation/ *Framework?*	• Education, training, and in-services.	45
	• Acceptance of evaluation was influenced by its basis on the *Framework*.	20
	• Direct involvement and discussion with staff.	20

ance companies). We attempted to overcome these challenges through education, peer support, in-services, student projects, and discussions. However, from ongoing research studies and chart review, we realized that staff require ongoing education and reorientation to the *Framework* process. Positive aspects of the evaluation identified were that the evaluation was client centered, occupation based, and functionally based and that the respondents enjoyed using the Occupational Profile. In accepting the new evaluation and the *Occupational Therapy Practice Framework: Domain and Process* (American Occupational Therapy Association, 2002; see Appendix K), respondents were influenced by education, training, in-services, and discussion with staff. Acceptance also was connected to the evaluation's basis on the *Framework* and thorough description of all occupational therapy areas to guide the profession's unique practice. Finally, respondents reported that their clinical practice had changed to be more client centered, occupation based, and holistic.

Client Outcomes

In March 2005, a survey was conducted to determine the clients' understanding of their goals and perceptions of occupational therapy services since the inception of the new documentation format. This survey was distributed to all occupational therapists at Cardinal Hill Rehabilitation Hospital for them to complete with clients during the discharge Occupational Profile. The survey consisted of four open-ended questions and was conducted for a 1-month period. Forty-nine surveys were returned, and all were included in the analysis. Clients were of varied ages with the following diagnoses: cerebrovascular accident, spinal cord injury, traumatic brain injury, sensory processing disorder, autism, and orthopedic conditions.

Mixed methods were used to analyze the data to calculate percentages and identify emerging themes. First, questionnaire results were analyzed, labeled, and cross-referenced to

Table 5.2. Clients' Responses to Occupational Therapy Outcomes

Survey Question	Major Theme Identified	% Respondents Identifying Theme (*N* = 49)
1. What were your occupational therapy goals when you first came to the hospital?	Various basic ADL goals	55
	Various IADL goals	23
	Walking	8
	Standing	6
2. Did you meet your occupational therapy goals?	Yes, I met my goals (some participants listed specific goals met).	76
	Goals were met partially.	22
	No, goals were not met.	2
3. How was occupational therapy different than your other therapies in helping you reach your goals?	Helped with BADL/IADL skills.	45
	OTs instilled confidence in me.	11
	I don't know.	8
	Increased my overall independence.	6
4. If you had to come here again, would you come to occupational therapy?	Yes, I would have occupational therapy again.	92
	Probably.	4
	I don't know.	2
	I would do whatever was required.	2

Note. ADL = activities of daily living; BADL = basic activities of daily living; IADL = instrumental activities of daily living; OT = occupational therapist.

develop categories. Categories were processed further, with additional information and examples added to each category until the categories reached a point of saturation. During this process, the constant-comparative method was used. This method consisted of constantly comparing labeled information to previous information to ensure that each piece of information was similar to all other information within the category. This process generated ideas, themes, and generalizations about each category (Bailey, 1997). Each of the four questions was analyzed individually. The results of this survey, which indicate that clients were able to identify a relationship between occupational therapy and activities of daily living, were aware of their individual goals, and were satisfied with the occupational therapy services they received, are presented in Table 5.2.

References and Bibliography

American Occupational Therapy Association. (1994). Uniform terminology for occupational therapy–Third edition. *American Journal of Occupational Therapy, 48,* 1047–1054.

American Occupational Therapy Association. (2002). Occupational therapy practice framework: Domain and process. *American Journal of Occupational Therapy, 56,* 609–639.

Bailey, D. M. (1997). *Research for the health professional: A practical guide* (2nd ed.). Philadelphia: F. A. Davis.

Beery, K. (1989). *Developmental Test of Visual–Motor Integration (Beery)–Revised.* Parsippany, NJ: Modern Curriculum Press.

Bruininks, R. (1978). *Bruininks–Oseretsky Test of Motor Proficiency.* Circle Pines, MN: Weston.

Cardinal Hill Rehabilitation Hospital. (2000, May). *Cardinal Hill policy and procedures.* Lexington, KY: Author.

Colarusso, R., & Hammill, D. (1996). *Motor-Free Visual Perception Test.* Novato, CA: Academic Therapy Publications.

Colman, W. (1992). Maintaining autonomy: The struggle between occupational therapy and physical medicine. *American Journal of Occupational Therapy, 47,* 63–70.

Dunn, W. (1981). *A guide to testing clinical observations in kindergarteners.* Rockville, MD: American Occupational Therapy Association.

Dunn, W., McIntosh, D. N., Miller, L. J., & Shyu, V. (1999). *Sensory Profile.* San Antonio, TX: PsychCorp.

Folio, M. R., & Fewell, R. R. (2000). *Peabody Developmental Motor Scales (PDMS–2).* Austin, TX: Pro-Ed.

Friedland, J. (1998). Occupational therapy and rehabilitation: An awkward alliance. *American Journal of Occupational Therapy, 52,* 373–380.

Gardner, M. (1996). *Test of Visual–Motor Skills–Revised.* Burlingame, CA: Psychological and Educational Publications.

Gentile, P. A. (2003, June). Overview of the *Occupational Therapy Practice Framework:* Part II. *Administration and Management Special Interest Section Quarterly, 19,* 1–4.

Harvison, N. (2003, March). Overview of the *Occupational Therapy Practice Framework:* Part I. *Administration and Management Special Interest Section Quarterly, 19,* 1–4.

Law, M., Baptiste, S., Carswell, A., McColl, M. A., Polatajko, H., & Pollock, N. (1994). *Canadian Occupational Performance Measure.* Toronto: Canadian Association of Occupational Therapists.

Nehring, A. D., Nehring, E. F., Bruni, J. R. Jr., Randolph, P. L., Sanford, A. R., Zelman, J. G., et al. (1992). *Learning Accomplishment Profile, Diagnostic edition.* Lewisville, NC: Kaplan Early Learning.

Paris, C., & Collins Boyle, D. (2005, June). Leadership in practice: Implementing the *Practice Framework* in a rehabilitation setting. *Administration and Management Special Interest Section Quarterly, 21,* 1–4.

Rogers, J., & Holm, M. (1994). Assessment of self-care. In B. R. Bonder & M. B. Wagner (Eds.), *Functional performance in older adults* (pp. 181–202). Philadelphia: F. A. Davis.

Schkade, J., & Schultz, S. (1992). Occupational adaptation: Toward a holistic approach for contemporary practice, Part I. *American Journal of Occupational Therapy, 46,* 829–836.

Schwartz, K. B. (1998). The history of occupational therapy. In M. E. Neistadt & E. B. Crepeau (Eds.), *Willard & Spackman's occupational therapy* (9th ed., pp. 854–860). Philadelphia: Lippincott-Raven.

Seidel, A. (1998). Theories derived from rehabilitation perspectives. In M. E. Neistadt & E. B. Crepeau (Eds.), *Willard & Spackman's occupational therapy* (9th ed., pp. 536–542). Philadelphia: Lippincott-Raven.

Taub, E., Crago, J. E., & McCulloch, K. L. (1997). *Arm Motor Activity Test (AMAT).* Unpublished instrument, Department of Psychology and Physical Therapy, University of Alabama at Birmingham.

Taub, E., & Wolf, S. L. (1997). Constraint-induced movement techniques to facilitate upper extremity use in stroke patients. *Topics in Stroke Rehabilitation, 3,* 38–61.

Uniform Data System for Medical Rehabilitation. (1997). *Guide for the uniform data set for medical rehabilitation* (Adult FIM; Version 5.1). Buffalo: State University of New York.

World Health Organization. (2001). *International classification of functioning, disability, and health (ICF).* Geneva, Switzerland: Author.

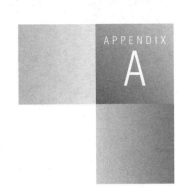

Cardinal Hill
Healthcare System
Occupational Profile
(Adult)

Cardinal Hill Healthcare System
Occupational Profile (Adult)

Client Name: _____ Client #: _____ DOB: _____

Initial Date: _____ Discharge Date: _____

Diagnosis: _____

Precautions: _____

1. Client lives ☐ with ☐ alone _____ in a ☐ house ☐ trailer ☐ apt. with _____ steps to enter ☐ R/ ☐ L handrail; _____ stories; _____ steps inside home. _____

   _____

2. Client's discharge environment, resources, and available adaptive equipment: _____

   _____

3. Prior to this hospitalization, the client was ☐ I ☐ min ☐ mod in BADLs and ☐ I ☐ min ☐ mod in IADLs. Client needed assistance with

   _____

   _____

4. A typical day consists of: wake up time _____ ☐ a.m. ☐ p.m.; ☐ volunteer ☐ work; bedtime _____ ☐ a.m. ☐ p.m.

   _____

   _____

   _____

   _____

   _____

5. What activities do you participate in for fun and how often? _____

6. How do you learn best? (In rehab you will be learning new things. Do you learn best by reading, watching a video?) _____

   _____

7. How familiar are you with technology? _____

8. What motivates you to improve? _____

9. How are you coping with your current status? _____

Initial Comments   **Discharge Comments**

List 5 occupations you want/need to resume	Satisfaction in resuming your roles

_____ _____   _____ _____
Therapist's Signature   Date   Therapist's Signature   Date

Note. R/L = right/left; I = independent; min = minimum; mod = moderate; BADLs = basic activities of daily living; IADLs = instrumental activities of daily living.

Cardinal Hill
Healthcare System
Occupational Analysis
(Adult)

Cardinal Hill Healthcare System
Occupational Analysis (Adult)

Client Name: _____ Client #: _____ DOB: _____

Initial Date: _____ Discharge Date: _____

Diagnosis: _____

Precautions: _____

Occupational Analysis:

Initial Comments   **Discharge Comments**

	Basic ADLs	
	Eating	
	Grooming	
	Bathing	
	E/W/S Dressing UB E/W/S	
	E/W/S Dressing LB E/W/S	
	Toilet TX	
	Tub/Shower TX	
	Problem Solving	
	Memory	
	Comments	

Note. This assessment form has been expanded to allow readers of all visual acuity to access its information. A 2-page form of this assessment can be found on the CD-ROM.

Page 1—Cardinal Hill Healthcare System Occupational Analysis (Adult)

Client Name: _____ Client #: _____

Initial Comments   **Discharge Comments**

	Instrumental ADLs	
	Community Mobility	
	Health Management	
	Home Management	
	Financial Management	
	Leisure	
	Safety	
	Comments	
	Movement Function	
	Sitting—Static/Dynamic	
	Standing—Static/Dynamic	
	Joint Stability and Skeletal Mobility	

Client Name: _____ Client #: _____

Initial Comments   **Discharge Comments**

	Place can on shelf	
	Retrieve item from floor	
	Screw lid on jar	
	Comb back of head	
	Write name	
	Lift grocery bag	
	Comments	

Client Name: _____ Client #: _____

Initial Comments   **Discharge Comments**

Initial Comments		Discharge Comments
	Energy for Task	
	Coordination	
L | | | R | |	Grip Strength/Lateral Pinch lbs/3 Jaw Chuck	L | | | R | |
	Knowledge/Organization of Task	
	Adaptation/Praxis	
	Comments	
	Social Interaction Skills	
	Cognitive & Affective	
	Level of Arousal/Attention	
	Orientation	
	Energy and Drive	

Page 4—Cardinal Hill Healthcare System Occupational Analysis (Adult)

Client Name: _____ Client #: _____

Initial Comments   **Discharge Comments**

Initial Comments		Discharge Comments
	Higher Level Cognition	
	Sensory	
	Visual	
	Perception	
	Pain	
	Skin Integrity	
	Comments	

	Pre	Post		Pre	Post		Pre	Post		Pre	Post		Pre	Post		Pre	Post
HR			O_2			RPD			HR			O_2			RPD			

Comments

Client Name: _____ Client #: _____

Initial Comments   **Discharge Comments**

How do the risks interfere with participation in occupation?	How has occupational therapy facilitated participation in occupation in client's environment?
Equipment:	Equipment provided:
	Goals met:
	Goals not met:
ELOS:	Number of visits:
	Reason for discharge:
	D/C recommendations/referrals:

_____   _____   _____   _____
Therapist's Signature   Date   Therapist's Signature   Date

Note. ADLs = activities of daily living; E/W/S = edge of bed/wheelchair/supine; UB = upper body; LB = lower body; TX = transfer; HR = heart rate; O_2 = oxygen; RPD = rate of perceived dyspnea; ELOS = estimated length of stay; D/C = discharge.

Page 6—Cardinal Hill Healthcare System Occupational Analysis (Adult)

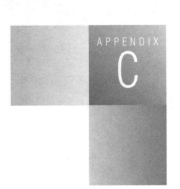

APPENDIX

C

Cardinal Hill
Healthcare System
Inpatient Intervention Plan

Cardinal Hill Healthcare System
Inpatient Intervention Plan

Client: _____ Client #: _____ DOB: _____

Admit Date: _____

Decreased satisfaction/ability to participate in the following occupations:

☐ Eating
☐ Grooming
☐ Bathing
☐ Dressing
☐ Toilet Transfer
☐ Tub/Shower Transfer

☐ Community Mobility
☐ Safety/Emergency Response
☐ Financial Management
☐ Health Management
☐ Home Management
☐ Social Participation

☐ Shopping
☐ Education
☐ Work
☐ Leisure/Play
☐ Functional Mobility

Performance risks that interfere with participation in occupations:

☐ Problem Solving
☐ Memory
☐ Cognition
☐ Posture
☐ Energy/Endurance
☐ Perception

☐ Neuromuscular/Movement
☐ Oral Motor/Dysphagia
☐ Mobility
☐ Coordination
☐ Strength/Effort

☐ Skin Integrity
☐ Pain
☐ Organization/Adaptability
☐ Sensory Functions
☐ Vision Functions

Strengths (contextual influences): _____

Short-term goals: _____

_____

_____

Discharge Goals/Rehab Potential: Client will demonstrate:

☐ 1. Eating with _____ using _____
☐ 2. Grooming with _____ using _____ ☐ w/c level ☐ walker level ☐ standing
☐ 3. Bathing with _____ using _____ ☐ sponge bath ☐ tub bath
☐ 4. Upper body dressing with _____ using _____ ☐ EOB ☐ w/c level ☐ supine
☐ 5. Lower body dressing with _____ using _____ ☐ EOB ☐ w/c level ☐ supine
☐ 6. Toilet transfer with _____ using _____ ☐ w/c level ☐ walker level
☐ 7. Tub/shower transfer with _____ using _____ ☐ w/c level ☐ walker level
☐ 8. Problem solving with _____
☐ 9. Memory with _____
☐ 10. Light homemaking activities with _____ using _____ ☐ w/c level ☐ walker level

Client/Family will:

☐ 11. Demonstrate knowledge to assist client with ADLs as needed
☐ 12. Perform home program with _____ assistance
☐ 13. Participate in community outing with _____ assistance ☐ w/c level ☐ walker level
☐ 14. Demonstrate use of equipment with _____ assistance
☐ 15. Engage in leisure exploration and/or participation with _____
☐ 16. _____
☐ 17. _____

Plan of Treatment/Education in:

☐ ADL	☐ Work/Productive Activities	☐ Psychosocial	☐ Positioning
☐ Neuromuscular Movement	☐ Cognitive Activities	☐ Sensory Activities	☐ Aquatics
☐ Skin/Edema	☐ Splinting/Casting	☐ Perceptual Tasks	☐ Leisure
☐ Modalities	☐ Oral Motor/Swallowing	☐ Re-Evaluation	☐ Co-Treat
☐ Adaptive Equipment	☐ D/C Planning	☐ Home Visit	☐ Other
☐ Home Program	☐ Client/Caregiver Education	☐ Home Safety/Equipment	

Frequency: _____ Duration: _____

Medical Diagnosis: _____

OT Diagnosis: _____

Contraindications/Precautions: _____

I certify that occupational therapy services are necessary under a plan to be periodically reviewed by me and while the patient is under my care.

_____	_____	_____	_____
Date	Therapist's Signature	Accepted Date	Physician's Signature

Note. w/c = wheelchair; EOB = edge of bed; ADLs = activities of daily living; D/C = discharge; OT = occupational therapist.

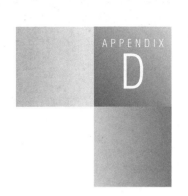

Cardinal Hill
Healthcare System
Outpatient Intervention Plan

Cardinal Hill Healthcare System
Outpatient Intervention Plan

Client: _____ Client #: _____ DOB: _____

Decreased satisfaction/ability to participate in the following occupations:

☐ Eating   ☐ Community Mobility   ☐ Shopping

☐ Grooming   ☐ Safety/Emergency Response   ☐ Education

☐ Bathing   ☐ Financial Management   ☐ Work

☐ Dressing   ☐ Health Management   ☐ Leisure/Play

☐ Toilet Transfer   ☐ Home Management   ☐ Functional Mobility

☐ Tub/Shower Transfer   ☐ Social Participation

Performance risks that interfere with participation in occupations:

☐ Problem Solving   ☐ Neuromuscular/Movement   ☐ Skin Integrity

☐ Memory   ☐ Oral Motor/Dysphagia   ☐ Pain

☐ Cognition   ☐ Mobility   ☐ Organization/Adaptability

☐ Posture   ☐ Coordination   ☐ Sensory Functions

☐ Energy/Endurance   ☐ Strength/Effort   ☐ Vision Functions

☐ Perception

Strengths (contextual influences): _____

Short-term goals: _____

_____

_____

_____

Discharge goals/rehab potential: _____

_____

_____

_____

Plan of Treatment/Education in:

☐ ADL   ☐ Work/Productive Activities   ☐ Psychosocial Skills   ☐ Positioning

☐ Neuromuscular   ☐ Cognitive Activities   ☐ Sensory Activities   ☐ Aquatics

☐ Skin/Edema   ☐ Splinting/Casting   ☐ Perceptual Tasks   ☐ Leisure

☐ Modalities   ☐ Oral Motor/Swallowing   ☐ Re-Evaluation   ☐ Co-Treat

☐ Adaptive Equipment   ☐ D/C Planning   ☐ Home Visit   ☐ HPOT

☐ Home Program   ☐ Client/Caregiver Education   ☐ Home Safety/Equipment   ☐ Other

Frequency: _____ Duration: _____

Medical Diagnosis: _____

OT Diagnosis: _____

Contraindications/Precautions: _____

I certify that occupational therapy services are necessary under a plan to be periodically reviewed by me and while the patient is under my care.

_____   _____   _____

Date   Occupational Therapist's Signature   Accepted Date

                          _____   _____

                                  Reviewing Physician's Signature   Reviewing Physician's Signature

                          _____   _____

                                  Reviewing Physician's Name   Referring Physician's Name

Note. ADLs = activities of daily living; D/C = discharge; HPOT = hippotherapy; OT = occupational therapist.

Cardinal Hill Healthcare System Protocol for Adult Occupational Therapy Evaluation, Long Form

Cardinal Hill Healthcare System
Protocol for Adult Occupational Therapy Evaluation,
Long Form

Occupational Profile

An occupational profile is defined as information that describes the client's occupational history and experiences, patterns of daily living, interests, values, and needs.

1. **Client lives (with, alone) _____ in (house, trailer, apartment) with _____ steps to enter (R/L handrail); _____ stories; _____ steps inside home.**
   Who is the client (e.g., individual, caregiver, group, population)? Collects information for determining client's roles (e.g., sibling). Determines *physical context* (i.e., nonhuman aspects of contexts). Includes the accessibility to and performance within environments having natural terrain, plants, animals, buildings, furniture, objects, tools, or devices (AOTA, 2002, p. 613).

   EVALUATION QUESTIONS
   - How many people besides yourself live in your home?
   - Do you live in a house, trailer, or apartment?
   - How many steps are at the entrance? Is your home all on one floor? If it's a two-story home, can all living be done on one floor?
   - Is there an easier access into the house, like a side entrance?
   - Is there a handrail present? Is it on the left or right as you are going up?

2. **Client's discharge environment, resources, and available adaptive equipment: _____.**
   Identify what equipment is present in the home. Determine future equipment needs and modification required for client and caregiver to be successful with occupational needs. This also may reveal other members in the home with risks, such as a spouse with back problems, and what caregiver support may be affected.

   EVALUATION QUESTIONS
   - Where will you go following discharge? How long?
   - Will you be alone any part of the day?
   - Do you have any equipment such as a tub seat, bath bench, elevated commode, rails, grab bars, handheld shower, long-handled sponge, sliding board? If equipment is present, do you use it?
   - Do you have magnifiers for low vision?
   - Do you have walk-in shower, standard tub, or tub/shower combination?

3. **Prior to hospitalization, client was (I, required assistance) in ADLs and (I, required assistance) in IADLs. Client needed assistance with _____.**
   Activities of daily living (ADL)
   Activities that are oriented toward taking care of one's own body (Rogers & Holm, 1994). See Analysis Protocol for detailed description of ADLs.

   Instrumental activities of daily living (IADL)
   Oriented toward interactions with the environment that are often complex and generally optional in nature.

   EVALUATION QUESTIONS
   - Did you need help with dressing, brushing your teeth, washing your face?
   - Were you able to perform activities such as running errands, housekeeping, bill paying, grocery shopping?
   - Did you drive prior to injury?

4. **A typical day consists of: wake-up time _____ (a.m., p.m.; volunteer; work), bedtime _____ (a.m., p.m.).**
   Temporal Context
   Location of occupational performance in time (e.g., stages of life, time of day, time of year, duration; AOTA, 2002, p. 613).

   Habits
   Useful Habits: Habits that support performance in daily life and contribute to life satisfaction. Habits that support ability to follow rhythms of daily life.

<u>Impoverished Habits:</u> Habits that are not established. Habits that need practice to improve.

<u>Dominating Habits:</u> Habits that are so demanding they interfere with daily life. Habits that satisfy a compulsive need for order.

Routines

Occupations with established sequences (Christiansen & Baum, 1997, p. 6).

Roles

A set of behaviors that have some socially agreed upon function and for which there is an accepted code of norms (Christiansen & Baum, 1997, p. 603).

<u>Care of Others (including selecting and supervising caregivers):</u> Arranging, supervising, or providing care for others.

<u>Care of Pets:</u> Arranging, supervising, or providing care for pets and service animals.

<u>Education:</u> Includes activities needed for being a student and participating in a learning environment.

<u>Formal Educational Participation:</u> Including the categories of academic (e.g., math, reading, working on a degree), nonacademic (e.g., recess, lunchroom, hallway), extracurricular (e.g., sports, band, cheerleading, dances), and vocational (pre-vocational and vocational) participation.

<u>Exploration of Informal Personal Educational Needs or Interests (Beyond Formal Education):</u> Identifying topics and methods for obtaining topic-related information or skills.

<u>Informal Personal Education Participation:</u> Participating in classes, programs, and activities that provide instruction/training in identified areas of interest.

<u>Work:</u> Includes activities needed for engaging in remunerative employment or volunteer activities (Mosey, 1996, p. 341).

<u>Employment Interests and Pursuits:</u> Identifying and selecting work opportunities based on personal assets, limitations, likes, and dislikes related to work (Mosey, 1996, p. 342).

<u>Employment Seeking and Acquisition:</u> Identifying job opportunities, completing and submitting appropriate application materials, preparing for interviews, participating in interviews and following up afterward, discussing job benefits, and finalizing negotiations.

<u>Job Performance:</u> Including work habits (e.g., attendance, punctuality, appropriate relationships with coworkers and supervisors, completion of assigned work, and compliance with the norms of the work setting; Mosey, 1996, p. 342).

<u>Retirement Preparation and Adjustment:</u> Determining aptitudes, developing interests and skills, and selecting appropriate avocational pursuits.

<u>Volunteer Exploration:</u> Determining community causes, organizations, or opportunities for unpaid work in relationship to personal skills, interests, location, and time available.

<u>Habits, Routines, and Roles</u>

EVALUATION QUESTIONS

- Can you walk me through a normal day, starting with the time you get up until you go to bed at night?
- What kind of work do you do? (If retired, what type of work did you do?) Do you plan to return to work, school, volunteer, etc.?
- What level of education did you complete? Can you read and write?
- How many days of the week do you follow this schedule? (Gives insight as to social patterns with community, family, peers.)
- Does this person interact with others, or is he or she alone the majority of the time?
- Does this person balance between work, play, and leisure activities?

<u>Care of Others</u>

EVALUATION QUESTIONS

- Do you care for anyone else besides yourself? What is your role?

<u>Care of Pets</u>

EVALUATION QUESTIONS

- Do you have pets?
- Who cares for your pets?
- What do you do if they're sick?
- Do you buy food, etc.?
- Do you walk your pets?

<u>Child Rearing</u>

EVALUATION QUESTIONS

- Do you have children/grandchildren/aunt or uncle, nephews/nieces?
- Do you play with your children/grandchildren? Describe an activity you might do with them.

Page 2—Cardinal Hill Healthcare System Protocol for Adult Occupational Therapy Evaluation, Long Form

Education

EVALUATION QUESTIONS

- Are you a student?
- What are your learning interests?

Work

EVALUATION QUESTIONS

- If you plan to return to work, how will you get to work?
- Do you work 8 hours per day?
- Will any accommodations be needed?
- Are you familiar with vocational rehabilitation services?

Retirement Preparation and Adjustment

EVALUATION QUESTIONS

- Do you have retirement plans?

5. **What activities do you participate in for fun, and how often?**
   Reveals information such as culture context (AOTA, 2002, p. 613).

   Cultural Context
   Customs, beliefs, activity patterns, behavior standards, and expectations accepted by the society of which the individual is a member. Includes political aspects, such as laws that affect access to resources and affirm personal rights. Also includes opportunities for education, employment, and economic support.
   Leisure and social participation will be addressed under the areas of occupation.

   Leisure
   "A nonobligatory activity that is intrinsically motivated and engaged in during discretionary time, that is, time not committed to obligatory occupations such as work, self-care, or sleep" (Parham & Fazio, 1997, p. 250).

   Social Participation
   Activities associated with organized patterns of behavior that are characteristic and expected of an individual or an individual interacting with others within a given social system (Mosey, 1996, p. 340).

   EVALUATION QUESTIONS

   - What were your prior interests?
   - Do you collect things?
   - Do you like to read about a topic?
   - Do you like to play games (computer or board)?
   - Do you go to church?
   - Do you go out to eat?

6. **How do you learn best? (In rehab you will be learning new things; do you learn best by reading, watching a video, etc.?)**
   See protocol for IADLs for further explanation in the area of education.

7. **How familiar are you with technology?**
   Relates to the *virtual* and *personal contexts*.

   Virtual Context
   Environment in which communication occurs by means of airways or computers and an absence of physical contact.

   Personal Context
   "Features of the individual that are not part of a health condition or health status" (WHO, 2001, p. 17). Personal context includes age, gender, socioeconomic status, and educational status.

   EVALUATION QUESTIONS

   - Do you have/use a computer?
   - Do you need anything to help you use the computer?

Page 3—Cardinal Hill Healthcare System Protocol for Adult Occupational Therapy Evaluation, Long Form

8. **What motivates you to improve?**

   Relates to the *personal* and *spiritual* and *cultural contexts* according to the *Framework*.

   Spiritual Context

   The fundamental orientation of a person's life; that which inspires and motivates that individual.

   Cultural Context

   Refer to definition above.

   Personal Context

   Refer to definition above.

   EVALUATION QUESTIONS

   - Why did you choose to come here?

   - Why do you want to get better?

   You may also include this information in the Client Factor Area under "Temperament and Personality Functions" as well as "Energy and Drive Functions."

9. **How are you/family coping with your current status?**

   (Also refers to *spiritual* and *cultural contexts*.)

   EVALUATION QUESTIONS

   - How are you handling this?

   - Are you anxious, depressed, positive?

10. **Occupation List**

    Initial: Identify 5 occupations you want/need to resume.

    1. _____

    2. _____

    3. _____

    4. _____

    5. _____

    May need to be completed after the analysis is completed and client has a good understanding of what occupational therapy is. The occupational therapist may help client with this section.

    This is a good time to redefine occupational therapy.

    This section drives the treatment plan and determines the goals for occupational therapy as determined by the client.

11. **At Discharge**

    You can rate the outcome or discharge response in this section with a satisfied or unsatisfied response. If the client is cognitively able, you may want to use a 1–10 scale to get a more exact response.

Basic Activities of Daily Living (BADL)

Activities that are oriented toward taking care of one's own body (Rogers & Holm, 1994); also called personal activities of daily living (PADL).

Eating/Oral Motor

Eating

The ability to keep and manipulate food and fluid in the mouth and swallow it (AOTA, 2000; O'Sullivan, 1995).

EVALUATION QUESTIONS

- Do you wear dentures?

- Can you cut all food and open containers?

- Can you locate all food items on tray?

- What is your motivation to eat food items?

Feeding
The process of setting up, arranging, and bringing food and fluids from the plate or cup to the mouth (AOTA, 2000; O'Sullivan, 1995).
FIM. Eating includes the ability to use suitable utensils to bring food to the mouth, as well as the ability to chew and swallow the food once the meal is presented in the customary manner on a table or tray. The client performs this activity safely.

Grooming
Obtaining and using supplies; removing body hair (use of razors, tweezers, lotions, etc.); applying and removing cosmetics; washing, drying, combing, styling, brushing, and trimming hair; caring for nails (hands and feet); caring for skin, ears, eyes, and nose; applying deodorant; cleaning mouth; brushing and flossing teeth; or removing, cleaning, and reinserting dental orthotics and prosthetics.
FIM. FIM scores based on following items (if valued by client then address option listed above): Grooming includes oral care, hair grooming (combing or brushing hair), washing the hands, washing the face, and either shaving the face or applying makeup. If the subject neither shaves nor applies makeup, grooming includes only the first four tasks. The client performs this activity safely. This item includes obtaining articles necessary for grooming.

Bathing
Obtaining and using supplies; soaping, rinsing, and drying body parts; maintaining bathing position; and transferring to and from bathing positions.

EVALUATION QUESTIONS
- What equipment do you use to bathe?
- When and how often do you bathe?
- Do you normally take showers or tub baths?
- Do you have a shower stall or tub/shower combination?

FIM. Bathing includes washing, rinsing, and drying the body from the neck down (excluding the neck and back) in a tub, shower, or sponge/bed bath. The client performs the activity safely.

Dressing Upper Body and Lower Body
Selecting clothing and accessories appropriate to time of day, weather, and occasion; obtaining clothing from storage area; dressing and undressing in a sequential fashion; fastening and adjusting clothing and shoes; and applying and removing personal devices, prostheses, or orthoses.
FIM—Upper Body. Includes dressing and undressing above the waist, as well as applying and removing a prosthesis or orthosis when applicable. The client performs this activity safely.
FIM—Lower Body. Includes dressing and undressing from the waist down, as well as applying and removing a prosthesis or orthosis when applicable. The client performs this activity safely.

EVALUATION QUESTIONS
- What equipment do you use to dress yourself?
- How long does it take you to dress?
- At home, do you sit at the edge of the bed or in a chair to dress yourself?

Transfers
Toilet Transfers
FIM. Toilet transfers include safely getting on and off a toilet.

Tub/Shower Transfers
FIM. Tub transfers include getting into and out of a tub. The client performs the activity safely.
FIM. Shower transfers include getting into and out of a shower. The client performs the activity safely.

Problem Solving
FIM. Problem solving includes skills related to solving problems of daily living. This means making reasonable, safe, and timely decisions regarding financial, social, and personal affairs, as well as the initiation, sequencing, and self-correcting of tasks and activities.

Memory
FIM. Memory includes skills related to recognizing and remembering while performing daily activities in an institutional or community setting. Memory in this context includes the ability to store and retrieve information, particularly verbal and visual. The functional evidence of memory includes recognizing people frequently encountered, remembering daily routines, and executing requests without being reminded. A deficit in memory impairs learning as well as performance of tasks.

Comments

Sexual Activity
Engagement in activities that result in sexual satisfaction.

Sleep/Rest
A period of inactivity in which one may or may not suspend consciousness.

EVALUATION QUESTIONS

- Do you take naps? Do you need medications to sleep?

Toilet Hygiene
Obtaining and using supplies; clothing management; maintaining toileting position; transferring to and from toileting position; cleaning body; and caring for menstrual and continence needs (including catheters, colostomies, and suppository management).

Functional Mobility
Moving from one position or place to another (during performance of everyday activities), such as in-bed mobility, wheelchair mobility, transfers (wheelchair, bed, car, tub, toilet, tub/shower, chair, floor). Performing functional ambulation and transporting objects.

Personal Device Care
Using, cleaning, and maintaining personal care items, such as hearing aids, contact lenses, glasses, orthotics, prosthetics, adaptive equipment, and contraceptive and sexual devices.

Instrumental Activities of Daily Living (IADL)

Activities that are oriented toward interacting with the environment and that are often complex and generally optional in nature (i.e., may be delegated to another; Rogers & Holm, 1994).

Community Mobility
Moving self in the community and using public or private transportation, such as driving or accessing buses, taxi cabs, or other public transportation systems.

EVALUATION QUESTIONS

- Do you drive?
- How do you get your errands done?
- Would you ride the bus or take a cab and know how?

For Home Care: Comment on client's homebound status.

Health Management and Maintenance
Developing, managing, and maintaining routines for health and wellness promotion, such as physical fitness, nutrition, decreasing health risk behaviors, and medication routines.

EVALUATION QUESTIONS

- What is your medication routine? How do you get your medications?
- Do you exercise?
- Do you plan to learn your medication routine? Would a medication organizer help?
- Do you adhere to the diet prescribed by your doctor?

Home Management
Obtaining and maintaining personal and household possessions and environment (e.g., home, yard, garden, appliances, vehicles), including maintaining and repairing personal possessions (clothing and household items) and knowing how to seek help or whom to contact.

EVALUATION QUESTIONS

- Do you cut the grass or shovel the snow?
- Can you repair broken items or change light bulbs?
- What would you do if you had a broken appliance?
- Do you do your laundry?
- Can you sew on a button?
- Do you clean your home?

Meal Preparation and Cleanup
Planning, preparing, and serving well-balanced, nutritional meals and cleaning up food and utensils after meals.

EVALUATION QUESTIONS

- Who cooks at home?
- What do you use to cook with?
- Do you plan your menu?
- What do you usually eat for dinner?
- Who does dishes?

Shopping
Preparing shopping lists (grocery and other); selecting and purchasing items; selecting method of payment; and completing money transactions.

EVALUATION QUESTIONS

- How do you grocery shop (make list, drive to, use coupons, read newspaper ads, etc.)?
- How do you pay?

Financial Management
Using fiscal resources, including alternate methods of financial transaction and planning, and managing finances with long-term and short-term goals.

EVALUATION QUESTIONS

- Who pays your bills?
- Who balances your budget?
- Do you have trouble seeing $ or ✓s?

Leisure
A nonobligatory activity that is intrinsically motivated and engaged in during discretionary time, that is, time not committed to obligatory occupations such as work, self-care, or sleep (Parham & Fazio, 1997).

Leisure Exploration
Identify interests, skills, opportunities, and appropriate leisure activities.

EVALUATION QUESTIONS

- What do you do for fun?
- Are you interested in learning other leisure tasks?
- Are there any barriers that would interfere with your participation in leisure tasks?

Leisure Participation
Planning and participating in appropriate leisure activities; maintaining a balance of leisure activities with other areas of occupation; and obtaining, using, and maintaining equipment and supplies as appropriate.

EVALUATION QUESTIONS

- Are there groups you would like to be involved with or rejoin (church activities, bowling league, bridge club, etc.)?

Play
Any spontaneous or organized activity that provides enjoyment, entertainment, amusement, or diversion (Parham & Fazio, 1997).

EVALUATION QUESTIONS

- What are your favorite toys?
- Who do you play with?

Play Exploration
Identifying appropriate play activities, which can include exploration play, practice play, pretend play, games with rules, constructive play, and symbolic play (Bergen, 1988).

Play Participation
Participating in play; maintaining a balance of play with other areas of occupation; and obtaining, using, and maintaining toys, equipment, and supplies appropriately.

Page 7—Cardinal Hill Healthcare System Protocol for Adult Occupational Therapy Evaluation, Long Form

Safety Procedures and Emergency Responses
Knowing and performing preventive procedures to maintain a safe environment as well as recognizing sudden, unexpected hazardous situations and initiating emergency action to reduce the threat to health and safety.

EVALUATION QUESTIONS
- If you have a fire that you can't control, what do you do?
- If you cut yourself, what do you do?
- If you fall, what do you do?
- How will you get out of your house in an emergency?

Comments
Further comments on IADLs.

Motor Skills (Movement Function)

Skills in moving and interacting with task, objects, and environment (A. Fisher, personal communication, July 9, 2001).

Posture
Relates to the stabilizing and aligning of one's body while moving in relation to task objects with which one must deal.

Stabilizes
Maintains trunk control and balance while interacting with task objects such that there is no evidence of transient (e.g., quickly passing) propping or loss of balance that affects task performance.

Aligns
Maintains an upright sitting or standing position, without evidence of a need to persistently prop during the task performance.

Positions
Positions body, arms, or wheelchair in relation to task objects and in a manner that promotes the use of efficient arm movements during task performance.

Mobility
Relates to moving the entire body or a body part in space as necessary when interacting with task objects.

Walks
Ambulates on level surfaces and changes direction while walking without shuffling the feet, lurching, instability, or using external supports or assistive devices (e.g., cane, walker, wheelchair) during the task performance.

Reaches
Extends, moves the arm (and when appropriate, the trunk) to effectively grasp or place task objects that are out of reach, including skillfully using a reacher to obtain task objects.

Bends
Actively flexes, rotates, or twists the trunk in a manner and direction appropriate to the task.

Coordination
Relates to using more than one body part to interact with task objects in a manner that supports task performance.

Coordinates
Uses two or more body parts together to stabilize and manipulate task objects during bilateral motor tasks.

Manipulates
Uses dexterous grasp-and-release patterns, isolated finger movements, and coordinated in-hand manipulation patterns when interacting with task objects.

Flows
Uses smooth and fluid arm and hand movements when interacting with task objects.

Strength and Effort
Pertains to skills that require generation of muscle force appropriate for effective interaction with task objects.

Moves
Pushes, pulls, or drags task objects along a supporting surface.

Transports
Carries task objects from one place to another while walking, seated in a wheelchair, or using a walker.

Lifts
Raises or hoists task objects, including lifting an object from one place to another, but without ambulating or moving from one place to another.

Calibrates
Regulates or grades the force, speed, and extent of movement when interacting with task objects (e.g., not too much or too little).

Grips
Pinches or grasps task objects with no "grip slips."

Process Skills

Energy
Refers to sustained effort over the course of task performance.

Endures
Persists and completes the task without obvious evidence of physical fatigue, pausing to rest, or stopping to "catch one's breath."

Paces
Maintains a consistent and effective rate or tempo of performance throughout the steps of the entire task.

Attends
Maintains focused attention throughout the task such that the client is not distracted away from the task by extraneous auditory or visual stimuli.

Neuromusculoskeletal and Movement-Related Functions

Functions of Joints and Bones
Mobility of joint functions: Passive range of motion.
Stability of joint functions: Postural alignment. *Note:* This refers to physiological stability of the joint related to its structural integrity as compared to the motor skill of aligning the body while moving in relation to task objects.
Mobility of bone functions: Frozen scapula, movement of carpal bones.

Muscle Functions
Muscle power functions: Strength.
Muscle tone functions: Degree of muscle tone (e.g., flaccidity, spasticity).
Muscle endurance functions: Endurance.

Movement Functions
Motor reflex functions: Stretch reflex, asymmetrical tonic neck reflex.
Involuntary movement reaction functions: Righting reactions, supporting reactions.
Control of voluntary movement functions: Eye–hand coordination, bilateral integration, eye–foot coordination.
Involuntary movement functions: Tremors, tics, motor preservation.
Gait pattern functions: Walking patterns and impairments, such as asymmetric gait, stiff gait. (*Note:* Gait patterns are assessed in relation to how they affect ability to engage in occupations and in daily life activities.)

Movement Function

Sitting/Standing–Static/Dynamic
Observe client's posture and mobility, his or her ability to stabilize and align him- or herself in relation to tasks for efficient use of UE.
Functional observation of client when bathing, dressing, grooming, bending, and reaching using the following scale:
Good (WFL): Able to sit/stand on flat surfaces without external or hand support
Modified independence: Client uses assistive device without supervision for balance while standing
Supervision (standby assist): Needs supervision to maintain balance to ensure safety
Minimal assistance (contact guard assist): Therapist provides 25% or less support to maintain balance
Moderate assistance: Therapist provides 26%–50% support to maintain balance
Maximum assistance: Therapist provides 51%–75% support to maintain balance
Total assistance: Therapist provides greater than 75% support to maintain balance

Joint Stability and Skeletal Mobility
Joint stability refers to the physiological stability of the joint related to its structural integrity as compared to the motor skill of aligning the body while moving in relation to task objects.

Note: shoulder subluxation, ulnar drift, nodules, Boutonniere deformity, Swan neck deformity, etc.

Measure shoulder subluxation according to finger distance between acromion and head of humerus. Mild = 1 finger; moderate = 1–2 fingers; severe = 3+ fingers

Skeletal mobility refers to the mobility of the bone.

Note: frozen scapula, movement of carpal bones, etc.

Performance Tasks

The following six tasks will be attempted and/or completed by the client in order to assess movement function. Some tasks may not be able to be assessed or performed secondary to visual or cognitive deficits, client precautions, or individual circumstances (e.g., client with a TLSO). Denote "unable to assess" or "not tested" and use an ROM or strength addendum if applicable. If client is able to perform task, denote "able" or "WFL." Then use the quality-of-movement scale and supplemental questions to further describe task performance. Use adaptive equipment to complete the tasks only if the client already has the adaptive equipment. Do not issue AE during the evaluation. Upon discharge, comment on AE issued and used to complete the tasks. Each unit has a performance task kit.

1. Place can on shelf:
* Note height of surface/type of surface (e.g., table)
* Note if client is sitting or standing

2. Retrieve item from floor:
* Use sock roll
* Note if client is sitting or standing

3. Screw lid on jar:
* Use peanut butter jar
* Lid should be tightened to the point it is not loose (i.e., snug)
* Note if client holds jar on table, on lap, or in mid-air
* Note which hand turns lid and how jar is stabilized

4. Comb back of head:
* Client can be sitting or standing
* Comb is held in right hand and transferred to left hand

5. Write name:
* Client is seated with paper positioned on a table of comfortable height in front of client, with forearm resting on table
* Client writes name with dominant hand; if unable because of motor deficits, nondominant hand is attempted

6. Lift a grocery bag (5 lb. bag of flour in bag):
* Client may be sitting or standing
* Note grasp pattern
* Note approximately how high client can lift bag (e.g., knee height, waist height, tabletop, etc.)

Quality-of-Movement Scale/Evaluation Questions

Not functional: No attempt made with involved arm. No movement initiated. Neglects involved extremity. Involved arm does not participate functionally; uninvolved arm may be used to move the involved extremity.

Stabilizer: Requires assistance of uninvolved extremity for minor readjustments or change of position, or accomplishes very slowly. In bilateral tasks, the involved extremity serves as a helper or stabilizer.

Gross assist: Movement is influenced to some degree by synergy or is performed slowly and/or with effort. Primitive grasp patterns may be present. May need cues to integrate extremity during task performance (e.g., uses involved limb to secure wheelchair lock with cues).

Functional: Movement is close to normal or appears to be normal; may be slightly slower; or lack precision, fine coordination, or fluidity.

EVALUATION QUESTIONS

Use the following questions to aid in making comments and describing the client's movement during task performance. Not all questions will be applicable or necessary to describe the movements. Comment on only those questions applicable and most important to establish baseline and discharge data.

During task performance, does the client
* Have adequate muscle tone bilaterally to perform task? Does the tone fluctuate during task performance? Note the type and/or degree of muscle tone (e.g., severe hypertonia).
* Have adequate joint mobility (AROM and PROM) bilaterally to perform task? Note limitations in AROM and PROM of joints involved in movement to complete task. Use percentages (%) to describe range of movement (e.g., client has 50% AROM of shoulder flexion).
* Have adequate strength and effort bilaterally to perform the task? Assign muscle grade if necessary (e.g., 3+/5 for elbow extension). Comment on how client moves, transports, lifts, and calibrates objects.

- Have adequate muscle endurance to complete the task (e.g., do muscles tire before the task is completed)?
- Have appropriate righting reactions, supporting reactions, eye–hand coordination, bilateral integration, and eye–foot coordination to complete the task?
- Present with substitution or synergistic movements while performing a task?
- Present with motor reflexes (e.g., ASTNR) or involuntary movements (e.g., tremors, tics, motor perserveration, or associated reactions) during task performance?
- Use a specific grasp pattern or an abnormal grasp pattern? Comment on the type of grasp pattern used (e.g., hook grasp, cylindrical grasp, power grasp). If abnormal, describe the grasp.
- Use adaptive equipment to complete the task (e.g., reacher, adapted utensils)?
- Use upper extremity as a stabilizer, gross assist, etc.? Refer to quality-of-movement scale for clarification.

Comments

Further comments on performance tasks and quality of movement as necessary.

Energy for Task

Sustained effort over course of task performance.

<u>Within functional limits:</u> Completes tasks without evidence of fatigue, rest break, or "catching breath" for 15 minutes or more, paces self maintaining a consistent effective rate. Heart rate within 20 beats of resting rate and/or SpO_2 level above 95.

<u>Fair:</u> Demonstrates fatigue, minimal shortness of breath, need for rest break during dressing, grooming, chair transfers, reaching into cupboards, moderate activity of less than 15 minutes, and/or SpO_2 level below 95.

<u>Poor:</u> Need for more than two rest breaks, moderate shortness of breath during 15 minutes or less of dressing, grooming, chair transfer, reaching into cupboards, moderate activity, and/or SpO_2 level below 90.

Coordination

Note WFL or impaired. Further comment on gross motor, fine motor, eye–hand, eye–foot, and bilateral integration. This line can be used for standardized tests or measures as necessary (e.g., 9 hole peg, box and blocks).

Hand Strength Tests

For each of the following tests of hand strength, the subjects will be seated with their shoulder adducted and neutrally rotated, elbow flexed at 90 degrees, forearm in neutral position and the wrist between 0 and 30 degrees dorsiflexion and between 0 and 15 degrees of ulnar deviation. For each strength test, the average of three successive trials will be the actual strength score. Grip strength will be measured by a standard adjustable handle dynamometer[1] set at the second handle position. It will be lightly held by the examiner around the readout dial to prevent inadvertent dropping. Pinch strength will be measured by a commercially available pinch gauge.[2] It will be lightly held by the examiner at the distal end to prevent dropping.

<u>Grip Strength:</u> "I want you to hold the handle like this and squeeze as hard as you can." Examiner demonstrates and then gives the dynamometer to subject. After subject is positioned appropriately, examiner says, "Are you ready? Squeeze as hard as you can." As client begins to squeeze, say "Harder! . . . Harder! . . . Relax." After the first trial score is recorded, the test is repeated with the same instructions for the second and third trial and for the other hand.

<u>Tip (Two Point) Pinch:</u> Tip Pinch is thumb tip to index finger tip. "I want you to place the tip of your index finger on this side as if to make an O. Curl your other fingers into your palm as I'm doing."

Examiner demonstrates the position and gives the pinch gauge to the subject. After the subject is positioned appropriately, the examiner says, "Are you ready? Pinch as hard as you can." As subject begins to pinch, say "Harder! . . . Harder! . . . Relax." After the first trial score is recorded, the test is repeated with the same instructions for the second and third trials and for the other hand.

<u>Key (Lateral) Pinch:</u> Key Pinch is thumb pad to lateral aspect of middle phalanx of index finger. "I want you to place your thumb on top and your index finger below as I'm doing and pinch as hard as you can." (Continue instruction as for Tip Pinch above.)

<u>Palmer (3 Jaw Chuck) Pinch:</u> Palmer Pinch is thumb pad to pads of index and middle fingers. "I want you to place your thumb on this side and your first two fingers on the side as I'm doing and pinch as hard as you can." (Continue instructions as for Tip Pinch above.)

<u>References</u>

Fess, E. E., & Moran, C. (1981). *Clinical assessment recommendations.* Chicago: American Society of Hand Therapists.

Kirkpatrick, J. E. (1956). Evaluation of grip loss: Factor of permanent disability in California. *California Medicine, 85,* 314–320.

Kraft, G., & Detels, P. (1972). Position of function of the wrist. *Archives of Physical Medicine, 53,* 272–275.

Mathiowetz, V., Weber K., Vollard G., & Kashman, W. (1984). Reliability and validity of grip and pinch strength evaluations. *Journal of Hand Surgery, 9,* 222–228.

---

[1]Jamar Dynamometer. Available from Asimow Engineering Co., Los Angeles, CA 90024.
[2]Pinch Gauge. Available from B & L Engineering, Santa Fe Springs, CA 90670.

Mathiowetz, V., Kashman, N., Vollard, G., Weber, K., Dowe, M., & Rogers, S. (1985). Grip and pinch strength: Normative data for adults. *Archives of Physical Medicine and Rehabilitation, 66,* 69–74.

Pryce, J. C. (1980). The wrist position between neutral and ulnar deviation that facilitates the maximum power grip strength. *Journal of Biomechanics, 13,* 505–511.

Compiled by Virgil Mathiowetz, MS, OTR
For additional information, send self-addressed stamped envelope to:
Virgil Mathiowetz, MS, OTR
University of Wisconsin, Milwaukee
Occupational Therapy Program
P.O. Box 413
Milwaukee, WI 53201
Phone: 414-963-5625 or -5615 (secretary)

The principal investigator would like to acknowledge the following people who assisted in various phases of this study. Many thanks to Karen Weber, Nancy Kashman, Gloria Volland, Mary Dowe, Sandra Rogers, Lori Donahoe, and Cheryl Rennells.

Knowledge and Organization

Knowledge
Seeking and using task-related knowledge.

Chooses
Selects appropriate and necessary tools and materials for the task, including choosing the tools and materials that were specified for use prior to the initiation of the task.

Uses
Uses tools and materials according to their intended purposes and in a reasonable or hygienic fashion, given their intrinsic properties and the availability (or lack of availability) of other objects.

Handles
Supports, stabilizes, and holds tools and materials in an appropriate manner that protects them from damage, falling, or dropping.

Heeds
Uses goal-directed task actions that are focused toward the completion of the specified task (i.e., the outcome originally agreed on or specified by another) without behavior that is driven or guided by environmental cues (i.e., "environmentally-cued" behavior).

Inquiries
(a) Seeks needed verbal or written information by asking questions or reading directions or labels or (b) asks no unnecessary information questions (e.g., questions related to where materials are located or how a familiar task is performed).

Organization
Organize space and objects as demonstrated in searching/locating materials in a logical manner.

Temporal Organization
Pertains to the beginning, logical ordering, continuation, and completion of the steps and action sequences of a task.
Initiates: Starts or begins the next action or step without hesitation.
Continues: Performs actions or action sequences of steps without unnecessary interruption such that once an action sequence is initiated, the individual continues on until the step is completed.
Sequences: Performs steps in an effective or logical order for efficient use of time and energy and with an absence of (a) randomness in the ordering and/or (b) inappropriate repetition ("reordering") of steps.
Terminates: Brings to completion single actions or single steps without perseveration, inappropriate persistence, or premature cessation.

Organizing Space and Objects
Pertains to skills for organizing task spaces and task objects.
Searches/locates: Looks for and locates tools and materials in a logical manner, including looking beyond the immediate environment (e.g., looking in, behind, above).
Gathers: Collects needed or misplaced tools and materials, including (a) gathering located supplies into the workspace and (b) collecting and replacing materials that have spilled, fallen, or been misplaced.
Organizes: Logically positions or spatially arranges tools and materials in an orderly fashion (a) within a single workspace and (b) among multiple appropriate workspaces to facilitate ease of task performance.

<u>Restores:</u> (a) Puts away tools and materials in appropriate places, (b) restores immediate workspace to original condition (e.g., wiping surfaces clean), (c) closes and seals containers and covers when indicated, and (d) twists or folds any plastic bags to seal.

<u>Navigates:</u> Modifies the movement pattern of the arm, body, or wheelchair to maneuver around obstacles that are encountered in the course of moving through space such that undesirable contact with obstacles (e.g., knocking over, bumping into) is avoided (includes maneuvering objects held in the hand around obstacles).

EVALUATION QUESTIONS

Can client

- Choose, use, and handle tools (ADL equipment) and materials for intended purposes with good hygiene and in an appropriate manner, protecting objects from damage or dropping?

- Heed using goal-directed actions without "environmental" distractions?

- Seek verbal or written information without asking unnecessary information?

- Initiate tasks without hesitation, sequence tasks in logical order with efficiency, and terminate tasks appropriately?

- Gather needed and misplaced materials?

- Organize tools in logical positions of use?

- Restore tools by putting way and cleaning up?

- Navigate using UE, movement patterns to maneuver around objects without disturbance?

Note: WFL or impaired and support with observations.

Adaptation/Praxis

Relates to the ability to anticipate, correct for, and benefit by learning from the consequences of errors that arise in the course of task performance.

Notices/Responds

Responds appropriately to (a) nonverbal environmental/perceptual cues (i.e., movement, sound, smell, heat, moisture, texture, shape, consistency) that provide feedback with respect to task progression and (b) the spatial arrangement of objects to one another (e.g., aligning objects during stacking). Notices and, when indicated, makes an effective and efficient response.

Accommodates

Modifies his or her actions or the location of objects within the workspace in anticipation of or in response to problems that might arise. The client anticipates or responds to problems effectively by (a) changing the method with which he or she is performing an action sequence, (b) changing the manner in which he or she interacts with or handles tools and materials already in the workspace, and (c) asking for assistance when appropriate or needed.

Adjusts

Changes working environments in anticipation of or in response to problems that might arise. The client anticipates or responds to problems effectively by making some change (a) between working environments by moving to a new workspace or bringing in or removing tools and materials from the present workspace or (b) in an environmental condition (e.g., turning on or off the tap, turning up or down the temperature).

Benefits

Anticipates and prevents undesirable circumstances or problems from recurring or persisting.

Praxis

Conceiving and planning a new motor act in response to an environmental demand.

U/A to carry out purposeful movement in presence of intact, sensation, movement, and coordination. Three types of apraxia: limb, constructional and dressing. Testing can be completed by oral command, imitation, or real objects.

<u>Dressing apraxia:</u> Result from constructional apraxia, unilateral neglect, and/or body scheme disorders. Observe functionally to determine cause between constructional neglect and body scheme disorders, then further evaluate as indicated.

<u>Limb apraxia</u>

a) Ideomotor: Able to carry out activity spontaneously but not on command. May be able to use objects but is clumsy.

b) Ideational: Difficulty with sequencing motor acts.

<u>Constructional apraxia:</u> The ability to build, construct, or put something together systematically.

EVALUATION QUESTIONS

Note: WFL or impaired and support with observations; also describe any apraxias.

Can client

- Relate to the ability to anticipate, correct for, and benefit by learning from consequences of errors that arise in course of task performance?

- Notice and respond appropriately to nonverbal environmental and perceptual cues (e.g., movement, sound, smells) and progress in task?

- Observe spatial arrangement of objects to one another, aligning objects as needed with effective and efficient response?
- Accommodate by modifying actions or location of objects in anticipation of problems that might arise?
- Change method/sequence of task?
- Change manner of tool use?
- Ask for assistance when needed?
- Adjust and anticipate response to problems that might arise, making appropriate changes?
  –Move in space?
- Use tools for intended purpose?
- Turn off water?
- Adjust temperature?
- Benefit – Anticipate and prevent undesirable circumstances from recurring or persisting?
  –Demonstrate home safety?
- Observe client for indications of difficulty with completing task on command, or dressing skills, using the following descriptions and definitions. Can client follow basic commands during ADL task and evaluation, ruling out motor deficits?
- *Functional Observations:* Difficulty with setting a table, making a sandwich, copying, drawing and constructing two and three dimensions.
- *Further Tests:*
  –Graphic: Copy geometric shape. Drawing without model (e.g., clock, house, flower).
  –Assembly: Three-dimensional block design.
- *Further Tests:*

  Test of intransitive (express feelings) limb apraxia:
  –Wave good-bye
  –Beckon "come here"
  –Finger on lip for "shh"
  –Signal "stop"

  Test of transitive (involve object use) limb apraxia:
  –Brush teeth
  –Shave your face
  –Hammer nail
  –Saw board
  –Use screwdriver

Social Interaction Skills

Refer to conveying intentions and needs and coordinating social behavior to act together with people (Forsyth & Kielhofner, 1999; Forsyth, Salamy, Simon, & Kielhofner, 1997; Kielhofner, 2002).

Communication Device Use
Using equipment or systems such as writing equipment, telephones, typewriters, computers, communication boards, call lights, emergency systems, Braille writers, telecommunication devices for the deaf, and augmentative communication systems to send and receive information.

Physicality
Pertains to using the physical body when communicating within an occupation.

Contacts
Makes physical contact with others.

Gazes
Uses eyes to communicate and interact with others.

Gestures
Uses movements of the body to indicate, demonstrate, or add emphasis.

Maneuvers
Moves one's body in relation to others.

Orients
Directs one's body in relation to others and/or occupational forms.

Postures
Assumes physical positions.

Information Exchange
Refers to giving and receiving information within an occupation.

Articulates
Produces clear, understandable speech.

Asserts
Directly expresses desires, refusals, and requests.

Asks
Requests factual or personal information.

Engages
Initiates interactions.

Expresses
Displays affect/attitude.

Modulates
Uses volume and inflection in speech.

Shares
Gives out factual or personal information.

Speaks
Makes oneself understood through use of words, phrases, and sentences.

Sustains
Keeps up speech for appropriate duration.

Relations
Relates to maintaining appropriate relationships within an occupation.

Collaborates
Coordinates action with others toward a common end goal.

Conforms
Follows implicit and explicit social norms.

Focuses
Directs conversation and behavior to ongoing social action.

Relates
Assumes a manner of acting that tries to establish a rapport with others.

Respects
Accommodates to other people's reactions and requests.

Social Participation
Activities associated with organized patterns of behavior that are characteristic and expected of an individual or an individual interacting with others within a given social system (Mosey, 1996).

Community
Activities that result in successful interaction at the community level (e.g., neighborhood, organizations, work, school).

Family
Activities that result in successful interaction in specific required and/or desired familial roles (Mosey, 1996).

Peer, Friend
Activities at different levels of intimacy, including engaging in desired sexual activity.

EVALUATION QUESTIONS
Comment on client's social interaction skills by using the following guidelines:
- Have you been able to go see family and friends or go out to dinner or shopping? Have you gone back to church or club activities?

- Does the client need anger management or conflict resolution training for healthier coping skills?
- Can the client express basic needs and wants? Does the client express him- or herself in writing, orally, etc.? Can client identify basic ADL items?

Observation Skills

EVALUATION QUESTIONS

- Does the client give eye contact?
- Is he or she able to maintain a conversation? For example, if the client has aphasia, how does he or she interact? With nods, yes/no, communication board or u/a and depend on family member or caregiver? Does he or she pick up facial expressions (e.g., TBI u/a to pick up social cues)?

Auditory Skills

EVALUATION QUESTIONS

- Does client have hearing aids, or is he or she hard of hearing in one or both ears?
- Does he or she use sign language?
- Is English the client's primary or secondary language?

Communication Device Use

EVALUATION QUESTIONS

- Are you able to use the phone, remote for TV?
- What do you do in an emergency (for D/C: lifeline device)?

Social Participation

EVALUATION QUESTIONS

- If you needed help, who would you call?
- Do you feel at this time you could socialize with your friends, family, and strangers?
- Does anxiety prevent you from participating in any occupations?

Cognitive, Affective

Global Mental Functions

Consciousness functions
Level of arousal, level of consciousness.

Orientation functions
To person, place, time, self, and others.

Sleep
Amount and quality of sleep. *Note:* Sleep and sleep patterns are assessed in relation to how they affect ability to effectively engage in occupations and in daily life activities.

Energy and drive functions
Motivation, impulse control, interests, values.

Specific Mental Functions

Attention functions
Sustained attention, divided attention.

Memory functions
Retrospective memory, prospective memory.

Thought functions
Recognition, categorization, generalization, awareness of reality, logical/coherent thought, appropriate thought content.

Page 16—Cardinal Hill Healthcare System Protocol for Adult Occupational Therapy Evaluation, Long Form

Energy and Drive

Motivation, impulse control, interest, values.

Higher Level Cognition

Judgment, concept formation, time management, complex problem solving, decision making.

Mental functions of language

Able to receive language and express self through spoken and written or sign language. *Note:* This function is assessed relative to its influence on the ability to engage in occupations and in daily life activities.

Calculation functions

Able to add or subtract. *Note:* These functions are assessed relative to their influence on the ability to engage in occupations and in daily life activities (e.g., making change when shopping).

Level of Arousal

EVALUATION QUESTIONS

- Comment on ease of arousal during ADL, note the amount of stimuli needed to arouse (stimulus—any sensory input including voice, touch, movement, cold, wet washcloth to the face). Note the time the client is able to maintain arousal level without reintroducing stimulus.

Attention Functions

EVALUATION QUESTIONS

- How much cueing does client need to attend during initial evaluation or ADL/IADL task?

- Note the amount of time client can attend to the task. Can client attend to one task (note the environment—whether it is busy/noisy versus calm/quiet)? Can client complete multiple-step tasks (note number of steps client is able to complete and again note the environment)? Also, comment on client's ability to attend during divided-attention tasks.

Orientation

EVALUATION QUESTIONS

- Observe client's ability to identify person, place, time, and situation.

- During ADL ask the client, "Where are you?" "What month is it?" "Why are you here?" etc.

Energy and Drive

EVALUATION QUESTIONS

- Values: See profile for valued ADLs and roles. Does the client appear motivated to complete ADLs such as grooming, dressing, etc., or does he or she want family or staff to do it instead? Is the client motivated to participate in therapy?

- Interest: See profile for what client wants to address here and when he or she goes home.

- Motivation: See Profile and Observation of ADLs. Interview client or family members to determine motivating factors and cooperation during therapies and completion of ADLs.

- Impulse Control: During ADL evaluate client's ability to control impulses. Note amount of physical cueing and/or verbal cueing used by the client to control impulsive behaviors.

- Energy and Drive, Higher Level Cognition: Can client perform routine/rote motor commands during basic ADL tasks? Can client perform non-routine/unfamiliar ADL tasks? Note how much cueing or modeling the client requires to complete the task.

- If unable to assess at admission, write "To Be Assessed" on the evaluation and complete during treatment.

- Refer also to financial management, home, and health maintenance.

- Can client take instructions learned during treatment and generalize them to ADL/IADL tasks? Is client realistic about injury/deficits and appropriate goals in rehabilitation? Can client find unfamiliar rooms in hospital (e.g., gift shop, vending machine) for topographical orientation?

- Can client perform non-routine/unfamiliar ADL tasks? Note how much cueing or modeling the client requires to complete the task. Can client perform check writing, money management tasks, medication regime, and meal planning (within dietary parameters)? Can client take instructions learned during treatment and generalize them to ADL/IADL tasks? Is client realistic about injury/deficits and appropriate goals in rehabilitation?

- Emotional functions: Can client regulate emotions in response to task at hand? Can client control his or her emotions?
- Self-esteem: Note client's confidence in abilities to participate in ADLs and ability to regain functional ADL abilities. Does the client make positive comments about self and abilities?

Sensory

Ability to perceive sensory input.

Sensory Stimulation

EVALUATION QUESTIONS

For each sensory stimulation item, comment on the following:

Type of Response
Note response as follows:
General Response (code GR): Client responds to stimuli in a nonspecific way.
Example: Light touch to arm produces total body movement; noxious stimuli produces trunk extension.
Localized Response (code LR): Client responds to stimuli in a specific way.
Example: With light touch to arm, client pushes object away or moves arm; noxious stimuli produces head turn toward object or an effort to push object away.
No Response (code NR): Client exhibits no response to presented stimuli.

Response Rate
Indicate approximate percentage of response to stimuli when this information is important.

Comments
Indicate when/how responses were elicited and any other sensory stimulation information that would assist in understanding and treatment of client.

Sensory functions related to temperature and other stimuli
Sensitivity to temperature, sensitivity to pressure, ability to discriminate temperature and pressure.

Tactile
Interpreting light touch, pressure, temperature, pain, and vibration through skin contact/receptors.

EVALUATION QUESTIONS

- Comment on how client responds to touch and temperature of washcloth.

Further test:
Light Touch: Touch client's arm, trunk, or face with a feather, piece of fur, or paint brush.
Deep Pressure: Stimulate client's arm with deep pressure from therapist's hand.
Pain: Pinch nail beds on hand and feet for recognition of pain on both right and left side.
Temperature: Use ice or hot/cold test tubes to test both upper extremities.

Tactile
Sensitivity to touch, ability to discriminate.

EVALUATION QUESTIONS

- Does client respond to temperature of water when grooming, look to extremity being touched?

Further test:
Light Touch: Lightly touch client's skin with fingertip or paint brush. Have client say "yes" or nod head each time stimulus is felt. For localization to touch, have client point to area touched.
Temperature: A tube of hot water and a tube of ice water are lightly placed on the client's arm in a random manner. The client is to state hot or cold when he or she feels a stimulus. (Hot=104°–113°; Cold=41°–50°; dried off before presentation.)
Sharp/Dull: Give instructions to the client. Begin the testing on an area of intact sensation, using point of safety pin for sharp and other end of safety pin for dull.
Semmes-Weinstein Monofilaments Test of Sensation: Start with monofilament number 2.83. Instruct the client to hold out hands in supinated position side by side. Instruct client to respond to sensation by moving the finger that was touched. Obstruct client's vision. Touch the monofilament to each finger (test monofilament "breaks") and hold for 1 1/2 seconds. Record the number of monofilament to which the client accurately responds including each finger/thumb. Indicate diminished sensation due to calluses. See key on evaluation form.

1.65 – 2.83 = WNL
3.22 – 3.61 = Diminished light touch
3.84 – 4.31 = Diminished protective sensation
4.56 – 6.45 = Loss of protective sensation
6.65   = Deep pressure sensation only

Two-Point Discrimination: The stimulus may be applied using a blunt-ended calibrated compass, Boley gauge, esthesiometer, or paper clip. The two points, separated by 2 mm, are applied along the longitudinal axis in the center of the zone to be tested. The two points are applied simultaneously and with equal, light pressure to the skin of the palmar surface of the palm and fingers. Heavy pressure invalidates the test by allowing the subject to perceive the two points when he would not be able to if correct pressure were used. One-point application trials are randomly interspersed with two points at 2 mm, the separation between the two points is increased by 1 mm.

Proprioception

Kinesthesia, joint position sense.

EVALUATION QUESTIONS

- Note client's response when upper extremity, lower extremity, and trunk are positioned.

- Does client position arms to brush hair or teeth? Does client know arm is off lapboard, or is client aware of laying on hemi-arm?

- One extremity is positioned by the evaluator and the client is asked to match the position with the other extremity; vision is occluded; one or more joints may be involved in the tested position. Also considered in proprioception testing can be the accuracy of the client's pointing response in the previous vision-occluded sensory tests.

Auditory

Hearing function. Response to sound. *Note:* This function is assessed in terms of its presence or absence and its affect on engaging in occupations and in daily life activities.

EVALUATION QUESTIONS

- Comment on how client responds to name, localization to sound.

Further test:
Response to Voice: Note how client responds when name is called throughout session; speak from left and right side of client.
Response to Music: Note how client responds to a variety of music types.
Noxious Noises: These may include loud hand clapping, rattling a jar of beans, ringing a bell; present from left and right.

Vestibular

Balance.

EVALUATION QUESTIONS

- Comment on how client responds when rolling, side-lying to sit, etc.

Further test:
Fast/Slow: Describe how client responds to different speeds of rolling, rocking.
Rock/Bounce: Describe how client responds to rocking, bouncing when in supine or sitting position.

Gustatory

Taste function; ability to discriminate tastes.

EVALUATION QUESTIONS

- Comment on how client responds to a variety of solids and liquids, to oral care—by opening mouth or munching. Any hypersensitivities?

Further test: Use a cotton swab to present the following stimuli to the client's mouth:
Pleasant: Fruit flavors
Noxious: Vinegar, peppermint

Olfactory

Smell function; ability to discriminate smell.
- Comment on whether client responds to smell of deodorant, soap, aftershave, or perfume with increased movement or localized response.

Page 19—Cardinal Hill Healthcare System Protocol for Adult Occupational Therapy Evaluation, Long Form

Further test: Note client's response to these types of stimuli presented in a small container or test tube and moved underneath client's nose.

Pleasant: Perfume, vanilla, fruit scents, etc.

Noxious: Ammonia, vinegar, etc.

Stimuli is presented for 1 second. Unaffected extremity should be evaluated first for a brief assessment. When testing dermatomes, see Spinal Cord Sensory Addendum (Appendix J). If client does not want to close his/her eyes, use a blindfold to occlude client's vision.

I: Intact, consistently able to respond correctly.

Mild: A few inconsistent or delayed responses are noted.

Moderate: 50% of responses are inconsistent, inaccurate, or delayed.

Severe: 75% of responses are inconsistent, inaccurate, or delayed.

Absent: Client unable to feel stimulus.

Unable: Client is unable to participate or understand instructions in order to give an accurate response.

Visual

Seeing functions; visual acuity, visual field functions.

EVALUATION QUESTIONS

- Recommend a vision screen for all neurological clients. If deficits present, evaluate further following this key.

- Comment on how client watches you when walking around the bed or talking about ADLs.

Further test:

Sudden Visual Stimuli: Note how client responds to object suddenly placed in field of vision.

Light/Dark: Note how client responds to suddenly turning on/off lights.

Familiar Picture: Note how client responds to a familiar picture placed in field of vision.

Acuity

EVALUATION QUESTIONS

- Does client, without trouble, recognize faces? Is print fuzzy or blurry, etc.?

Further test:

Near: Snellon Vision Card place 14" from client's eyes. Client reads largest line first, moving downward. Examiner notes smallest line client can read in entirety or the line in which less than half the letters are missed. If 20/100 or less, then record that the client has difficulty reading small print.

Far: Client stands/sits 20' from chart and reads rows of letters down the chart. Scoring is the same as Snellon Near testing above.

Ocularmotor Control

EVALUATION QUESTIONS

- Does client complain of double vision; does he or she squint, blink excessively, resist head change, etc.?

Further test:

Ocular Pursuits/Tracking: The client is asked to track a moving object to assess quality-of-eye movement. Examiner holds object 12"–16" from client's eyes, moving it slowly in vertical, horizontal, and diagonal patterns. Client is instructed to "move just your eyes, not your head." Assess tracking ability can be done simultaneously with range-of-motion evaluation.

Rating scale:

Intact: Client moves eyes smoothly with no jerkiness, able to maintain fixation with no head movement.

Impaired: Eye movement is not smooth; client is unable to maintain fixation on object on one or both sides; client is unable to isolate head from eye movement; eye movement is slower to the involved side.

Convergence/Divergence

Medial and lateral rotation of eyes, which causes the lines of vision of the two eyes to meet on the target. Hold a bright object approximately 18" away from client's eyes; slowly move inward toward eyes, noting medial rotation of eyes. The closest point the client can fixate on target with both eyes is the convergence near point (CNP).

Rating scale:

Intact: Smooth, symmetrical medial rotation of both eyes up to approximately 9"–12".

Impaired: Asymmetrical movement on one or both eyes, CNP >12 inches.

Saccades

Two brightly colored objects are held 12"–18" from client's eyes, approximately 12" apart. Client is asked to look back and forth, from one object to the other, on demand. Examiner then changes the position of the objects, as client attends to the opposite object.

Rating scale:

Intact: Rapid, smooth, localization/fixation on target (slight under- or overshooting is normal).

Impaired: Under- or overshooting; long delay in fixating on object (>1 second); inability to isolate head and eye movement; jerky eye movements.

Eye Alignment

If client complains of double vision despite adequate ROM, ocular alignment should be assessed further. Perceiving a single visual image is dependent on both eyes receiving an image of an object on the corresponding retinal area of each eye. If the visual image falls on the fovea of one eye but not the other, a double image may be perceived.

Corneal Reflection Test

In dimly lit room, hold a penlight vertically under client's nose, so as to shine a reflection into each eye. A reflection off cornea in each eye should be observed, symmetrically placed in each eye, relative to the pupil.

Rating scale:

Intact: Symmetrical reflections relative to pupil in left and right eye.

Impaired: Asymmetrical reflections (e.g., one reflection in center of pupil, one to left of pupil).

Cover/Cross Cover Test

Client asked to fixate at examiner's nose, slightly lateral to midline. Without telling client in advance, quickly cover one eye with small card or paper (index card), moving it from chin upward in front of eye. Notice any movement of uncovered eye. Repeat on opposite eye.

Rating scale:

Intact: No movement of uncovered eye.

Impaired: Uncovered eye moves to fixate on object.

Visual Fields

Quantity of Vision—When eyes are in straightforward position, normal visual fields are approximately 64° upward, approximately 75° downward, approximately 60° inward, and approximately 90° outward. Total visual field is approximately 80° wide. Perimeter testing is available through an ophthalmologist and should often be pursued. However, informal visual field testing can be completed in the following manner:

EVALUATION QUESTIONS

- Does client start to one side, stay close to a wall when navigating, brush one side of head or teeth, etc.?

Confrontation

Examiner stands behind the client, and a second person sits directly in front of the client. The client is asked to focus on a target 12"–18" from the client's eyes (could be examiner's nose). The examiner moves a dowel with a white tip from outside the visual fields toward midline (from the left, right, superior, and inferior positions). At least 10–15 passes of dowel are generally necessary to obtain adequate information about visual fields. Examiner notes deviations from standards listed above.

Rating scale:

Intact: Client's visual fields correspond with examiner's (assuming examiner's are normal) or are within 30% of visual fields listed above.

Impaired: Client's visual fields are at least 30% less than examiner's (assuming examiner's are normal) or norms listed above.

Attention/Scanning

Visual scanning is a motor activity driven by attention, both attention and scanning occurring simultaneously. Normal visual scanning occurs in very organized and efficient ways.

EVALUATION QUESTIONS

- Comment on client's ability to navigate on unit, locate grooming items at sink, etc.

Intrapersonal Space—Within 20" of trunk

Scanning with Structured Array—Consider using letter-cancellation task. Place paper on table at client's midline. Ask client to cross out specified letter or symbol on paper. Examiner notes time needed to complete, pattern of scanning (as seen in the order of items crossed out), attention to detail throughout, symmetry in left and right performance. If client is unsuccessful, examiner provides strategy for success, such as using left-to-right scanning pattern, use of hand to lead visual search, use of anchor, etc. Examiner notes client's success with adaptive strategy.

Rating scale:

Intact: Client uses organized, structured approach (e.g., left to right, top to bottom) and misses no details on left or right, within reasonable time.

Impaired: Client omits characters and uses a random, disorganized approach to scanning. Note client's ability to use compensatory strategies. Clients with visual field loss without an attention and/or scanning deficit may take up to 7 minutes to complete cancellation task, but are able to use organized strategies and scanning patterns to do so.

Scanning With Unstructured Array

Line Bisection Test—In Line Bisection Test, client is asked to mark the center point on each of the horizontal lines on the page.
Rating scale:

Intact: If Line Bisection Test used, client should be able to mark center of horizontal lines within 1 cm.

Impaired: In Line Bisection Test, client unable to mark center of lines within 1 inch. Client unable to attend to detail.

Homonymous Hemianopsia

Blindness of right-sided or left-sided vision of both eyes.

Testing

The therapist sits facing the client. The individualized colored blocks are randomly placed (a minimum of two to each side) on the client's shoulder. Instructions are given: "You are allowed to turn your head. What color do you see?" (If aphasic, have client identify colors placed in front of him or her.) The client then responds verbally.

Color-Blind

Absence of or defect in the perception of colors. The most common class of color-blindness is based on the perception of red, green, and blue (termed the 1st, 2nd, and 3rd color factors, respectively). Color-blindness in which all colors are perceived as gray is termed *monochromasia.*

Glasses

Comment if client has glasses or not.

Perception

Visuospatial perception, interpretation of sensory stimuli (tactile, visual, auditory, olfactory, gustatory).

Body Image

EVALUATION QUESTIONS

- Note client's ability to perform task with awareness of body scheme and R/L discriminate.
- Note amount of physical cueing and/or verbal cueing needed to attend to affected body parts.
- Note awareness client has of deficits in body scheme and body image.
- Does client follow body commands during ADLs?
- Does client follow body part commands in ADLs?

Self-concept

EVALUATION QUESTIONS

- Can client identify strengths and weaknesses about him- or herself?
- Does the client put him- or herself down frequently or make "I" statements?
- Does the client appear inflexible or resistant to trying adaptive technique?
- Does the client appear demanding of the therapist to assist in ADLs in a certain manner?
- Does the client appear positive and confident in his or her ability to regain skills in the future?

Experience of self and time functions

EVALUATION QUESTIONS

- Is the client aware of all body parts (note _____, etc.)?
- Does the client display appropriate self-concept; is he or she aware of change since the injury?
- Does client make appropriate positive comments about self, or does he or she make inappropriate negative comments?

Figure Ground

Differentiating between foreground and background forms and objects.

EVALUATION QUESTIONS

Observe if client can complete the following:
- Find towel and/or washcloth on bed (same color)?
- Find ADL items located at sink?
- Find eyeglasses, etc., in cluttered drawer?
- Does client have trouble finding the sleeve of unicolor shirt?
- Find wheelchair lock?

Further test:
In drawer, client points to four grooming items (comb, deodorant, toothpaste, toothbrush, towel, washcloth, etc.)
Scoring:
Intact: Client points to 4 items within 10 seconds per item.
Impaired: Client points to 0–3 items, or response is greater than 10 seconds.
Further test: MVPT, VOSP

Depth Perception
Determining the relative distance between objects, figures, or landmarks and the observer, and changes in planes of surfaces.

EVALUATION QUESTIONS

Observe if client can complete the following:
- Put toothpaste on toothbrush.
- Pour water into glass.
- Put glasses on.
- Put washcloth in water stream.
- Position wheelchair for transfer.

Scoring:
Intact: Client correctly completed 2 of the examples.
Impaired: Client responds correctly 0–1 time, or response is greater than 10 seconds.
Further Test: None

Pain

A basic bodily sensation induced by a noxious stimulus.

EVALUATION QUESTIONS

- Note client's painful reactions with movement; observe for facial grimaces, withdrawals.
- Ask client if he/she presently has pain and location of pain.
- Have client describe sensation of pain (e.g., dull, stabbing).
- Have client rate pain on 1–10 scale, 1 being lowest and 10 being highest.

Skin Integrity

Protective Functions of the Skin
Presence or absence of wounds, cuts, or abrasions.

Repair Function of the Skin
Wound healing.

Hair and Nail Functions
Occupational therapists and occupational therapy assistants have knowledge of these body functions and understand broadly the interaction that occurs between these functions and engagement in occupation to support participation. Some therapists may specialize in evaluating and intervening with a specific function as it is related to supporting performance and engagement in occupations and activities targeted for intervention.

Wounds
- Bleeding, depth, drainage, exposed anatomical structures location, odor, pigment, shape, size, staging: progression, tunneling
- Digital and grid measurements, grading of sores, observations, palpations, photographic assessments: wound tracing
- Signs of infection
- Wound scar tissue: banding, pliability, sensation and tecture scar rating scales
- Note activities, positioning, and postures that aggravate the wound or scar or that produce or relieve trauma

Associated Skin
- Blistering, continuity of skin color, dermatitis, hair growth, mobility, temperature, texture, turgor
- *Note:* Assistive, adaptive, orthotic, protective, supportive, or prosthetic devices and equipment that may produce or relieve trauma to the skin
- *Note:* General observations

Edema
- Note edema if hand size appears unequal. If appears equal, record "no significant edema noted," or if edema control is a goal, objective measure should be recorded using a volumeter or a circumferential measure.

Tests
Hand Volumeter: Set to measure hand and distal forearm edema. Fill the volumeter tank to the highest level/slight overflow. Place the overflow receiving pail under the volumeter immersion. Instruct the client to immerse the one hand into the volumeter tank with fingers three and four (long finger and ring finger) straddling horizontal bar near base of tank. Note measurements by transferring displaced water from pan into the 500 ml graduated cylinder. Note precise measurement in cylinder. Note edema by comparing amount of water displaced by each hand/distal forearm measurement.
Circumferential Measurements: Use plastic tape with respect to anatomical landmarks. Accuracy and reliability depend on consistency of tape placement and tension applied when pulling tape.
Guidelines: 10 cm. up/down from lateral epicondyle, over, ulnar styloid, MCP, DIP, PIP, dorsal of hand.

Comments

Psychomotor Functions
Appropriate range and regulation of motor response to psychological events.

Emotional Functions
Appropriate range and regulation of emotions, self-control.

Experience of Self and Time Functions
Body image, self-concept, self-esteem.
Psychomotor functions: Does the client display any inappropriate motor behaviors in response to psychological events? Does the client act out physically during event, or is client able to control motor use in relation to event?
Emotional functions: Can client regulate emotions in response to task at hand? Can client control his or her emotions?
Sleep: Note client's routine sleep cycle prior to and after injury/insult. Is the client's sleep pattern quality or not? Does client have day/night reversed?
Temperament/personality functions: What was the client's temperament or personality prior to injury? Note changes in personality post-injury. How does client's emotional state impact ADL/IADL participation?
Mental functions at language: Can client follow basic commands during ADL task and evaluation, ruling out motor deficits? Can client express basic needs and wants? Does the client express his/herself in written or verbal format? Can client identify basic ADL items?

Cardiovascular and Respiratory Functions

Blood Pressure Functions
Hypertension, hypotension, postural hypotension.

Hematological and Immunological System Function
Occupational therapists and occupational therapy assistants have knowledge of these body functions and understand broadly the interaction that occurs between these functions and engagement in occupation to support participation. Some therapists may specialize in evaluating and intervening with a specific function as it is related to supporting performance and engagement in occupations and activities targeted for intervention.

Respiration functions
Rate, rhythm, and depth.

Additional Functions and Sensations of the Cardiovascular and Respiratory Systems
Exercise tolerance functions: Physical, endurance, aerobic capacity, stamina, and fatigability.

EVALUATION QUESTIONS

- What medications are you on?

- Have you had heart surgery or high blood pressure?

- Do you have trouble breathing, especially when bathing or dressing or going up steps?

RPD = Rate of Perceived Dyspnea (How does client rate the difficulty with breathing while performing activities, ADLs, and IADLs?) Also known as Borg Scale 0–10

S02 = >95%

If S02 is <90%, have client sit and PLB

PLB = Pursed lip breathing   *DB* = Diaphragmatic breathing

0 = Nothing at all

0.5 = Very, very slight (just noticeable)

1 = Very slight

2 = Slight

3 = Moderate

4 = Somewhat severe

5 = Severe

6 = More severe

7 = Very severe (must rest)

8 =

9 = Very, very severe

10 = Maximal (must stop activity)

Cardiac Protocol Formula: max HR = 220 − age

0.5 to 0.75 (max HR − RHR) + RHR

Other Areas to Consider From the *Practice Framework*

[To be noted in comments as appropriate]

Occupational therapists and occupational therapy assistants have knowledge of these body functions and understand broadly the interaction that occurs between these functions and engagement in occupation to support participation. Some therapists may specialize in evaluating and intervening with a specific function as it is related to supporting performance and engagement in occupations and activities targeted for intervention.

- Voice and speech functions

- Digestive, metabolic, and endocrine system function

- Digestive system function

- Metabolic system and endocrine system function

- Genitourinary and reproductive functions

- Urinary functions

- Genital and reproductive functions

- Structure of the nervous system

- The eye, ear, and related structures

- Structures involved in voice and speech assistants

- Structures of the cardiovascular, immunological, and respiratory systems

- Structures related to digestive performance

- Structures related to the genitourinary and reproductive systems

- Structures related to movement

- Skin and related structures

Risks That Interfere With Participation of Occupation

Initial (eval) (protocol)

How do risks interfere with participation?

How do the client's performance areas, skills, patterns, context, activity demands, and client factors interfere with his or her ability to participate in occupation? Base your report on client's goals and priorities based on the environment he or she will be living in.

Page 25—Cardinal Hill Healthcare System Protocol for Adult Occupational Therapy Evaluation, Long Form

How Has Occupational Therapy Facilitated Participation in Occupation in the Client's Environment?

Discharge (eval) (protocol)

How has occupational therapy facilitated participation in occupation in client's environment?

How did client benefit from your treatment, so that he or she may generalize what he or she learned to other environments (include home program, family teaching, adaptive equipment, assistive technology, and community resources that increase client's success)?

Equipment

Comment on equipment client had before admission, provided during admission, and equipment that is being recommended.

ELOS

Comment on expected length of stay for client.

Goals Met

Identify which goals from treatment plan the client met during admission.

Goals Not Met

Identify which goals from treatment plan the client did not meet and why.

Number of visits

For COS indicate the number of times the client attended therapy.

Reason for Discharge

Indicate reason for client discharge.

Discharge recommendations/referrals

Indicate the recommendations for client upon discharge and where the client was referred.

Therapist Signature and Date

Therapist must sign evaluation and put date completed.

References

American Occupational Therapy Association. (2000). Specialized knowledge and skills for eating and feeding in occupational therapy practice. *American Journal of Occupational Therapy, 54,* 629–640.

American Occupational Therapy Association. (2002). Occupational therapy practice framework: Domain and process. *American Journal of Occupational Therapy, 56,* 609–639.

Bergen, D. (Ed.). (1988). *Play as a medium for learning and development: A handbook of theory and practice.* Portsmouth, NH: Heinemann Educational Books.

Forsyth, K., & Kielhofner, G. (1999). Validity of the assessment of communication and interaction skills. *British Journal of Occupational Therapy, 62,* 69–74.

Forsyth, K., Salamy, M., Simon, S., & Kielhofner, G. (1997). *Assessment of communication and interaction skills.* Chicago: University of Illinois, Model of Human Occupation Clearinghouse.

Kielhofner, G. (2002). Dimensions of doing. In G. Kielhofner (Ed.), *A model of human occupation: Theory and application* (3rd ed.). Philadelphia: Lippincott Williams & Wilkins.

Mosey, A. C. (1996). *Applied scientific inquiry in the health professions: An epistemological orientation* (2nd ed.). Bethesda, MD: American Occupational Therapy Association.

O'Sullivan, N. (1995). *Dysphagia care: Team approach with acute and long-term patients* (2nd ed.). Bollingbrook, IL: Sammons Preston.

Parham, L. D., & Fazio, L. S. (Eds.) (1997). *Play in occupational therapy for children.* St. Louis, MO: Mosby.

Rogers, J., & Holm, M. (1994). Assessment of self-care. In B. R. Bonder & M. B. Wagner (Eds.), *Functional performance in older adults* (pp. 181–202). Philadelphia: F. A. Davis.

World Health Organization. (2001). *International classification of functioning, disability, and health (ICF).* Geneva, Switzerland: Author.

Note. R/L = right/left; ADL = activities of daily living; I = independent; IADL = independent activities of daily living; BADL = basic activities of daily living; PADL = personal activities of daily living; UE = upper extremity; WFL = within functional limits; u/a = unable; TBI = traumatic brain injury; D/C = discharge; WNL = within normal limits; CNP = convergence near point; cm = centimeter; MCP = metacarpal phalangeal joints; DIP = distal interphalangeal joints; PIP = proximal interphalangeal joints; PLB = pursed lip breathing; DB = diaphragmatic breathing; HR = heart rate; RHR = resting heart rate; ROM = range of motion; TLSO = thoracic lumbar sacral orthotic; AROM = active range of motion; PROM = passive range of motion; AE = adaptive equipment; ASTNR = asymmetrical tonic neck reflex; ELOS = expected length of stay; COS = Center for Outpatient Services.

Cardinal Hill
Healthcare System
Protocol for Adult
Occupational Therapy
Evaluation, Short Form

Cardinal Hill Healthcare System
Protocol for Adult Occupational Therapy Evaluation,
Short Form

Occupational Profile

1.
- How many people besides yourself live in your home?
- Do you live in a house, trailer, apartment?
- How many steps to enter? Is your home all on one floor? If a two-story home, can all living be done on one floor?
- Is there an easier access into the house like a side entrance?
- Is there a handrail present? Is it on the left or right as you are going up?

2.
- Where will you go following discharge? How long?
- Will you be alone any part of the day?
- Do you have any equipment such as a tub seat, bath bench, elevated commode, rails, grab bars, hand-held shower, long-handled sponge, sliding board? If equipment is present, do you use it?
- Do you have magnifiers for low vision?
- Do you have walk-in shower, standard tub, or tub-shower combination?

3.
- Did you need help with dressing, brushing your teeth, washing your face?
- Were you able to perform activities such as running errands, housekeeping, bill paying, grocery shopping? Did you drive prior to injury?

4.
- Can you walk me through a normal day starting with the time you get up until you go to bed at night?
- What kind of work do you do? (If retired, what type of work did you do?) Do you plan to return to work, school, volunteer, etc.?
- What level of education did you complete? (Can you read and write?)
- How many days of the week do you follow this schedule?
- Does this person interact with others or are they alone the majority of the time?
- Does this person balance between work, play, and leisure activities?
- Do you have pets? Who cares for your pets? What do you do if they're sick? Do you buy food, etc.? Do you walk your pets?
- Are you a student? What are your learning interests?
- If you plan to return to work, how will you get to work? Do you work 8 hours per day, etc.? Will any accommodations be needed? Are you familiar with voc rehab services?
- Do you have retirement plans?

5.
- What were your prior interests?
- Do you collect things?
- Do you like to read about a topic?
- Do you like to play games (computer or board)?
- Do you go to church?
- Do you go out to eat?

6.
- Do you learn best when something is demonstrated or verbally described to you?
- Would you like to see pictures of tasks before you do them?
- Is watching a video more effective for your learning?

7.
- Do you have/use a computer?
- Do you need anything to help you use the computer?

8.
- Why did you choose to come here?
- Why do you want to get better?

9.
- How are you handling this?
- Are you anxious, depressed, positive?
- Comment if client is labile, etc.

10. Occupation List
- Initial: Identify 5 occupations you want or need to resume.
- At discharge: Rate the outcome or discharge response in this section with a satisfied or unsatisfied response. If the client is cognitively able, you may want to use a 1–10 scale to get a more exact response.

Basic Activities of Daily Living (BADLs)

Eating
- Does client wear dentures?
- Can client cut all food and open containers?
- Can client locate all food items on tray?
- What is client's motivation to eat food items?

Grooming
- Can client obtain grooming supplies?
- Can client groom self?
- Does client wear makeup or want to shave?
- Does client want to trim nails or floss teeth?
- Can client apply deodorant?

Bathing
- What equipment does client use to bathe?
- When and how often does client bathe?
- Does client normally take showers or tub baths?
- Does client have a shower stall or tub/shower combination?

Dressing UB and LB
What equipment do you use to dress yourself? How long does it take you to dress? At home, do you sit at the edge of the bed or in a chair to dress yourself?

Toilet Transfers
- Can client transfer self to toilet similar to type that he or she will use at home?

Tub/Shower Transfers
- Can client transfer self into bath or onto tub bench?
- What type of tub/shower does client have at home?

Problem Solving
- Can client adjust self and situation if problem arises?

Memory

Comments
- Does client take naps or medications to sleep?

Instrumental Activities of Daily Living (IADLs)
Community Mobility
- Do you drive?
- How do you get your errands done?
- Would you ride the bus or take a cab and know how?

For home care: Comment on client homebound status

Health Management and Maintenance
- What is your medication routine?
- How do you get your meds?
- Do you exercise?
- Do you plan to learn your medication routine?
- Would a med organizer help?
- Do you adhere to the diet prescribed by your doctor?

Home Management
- Do you cut the grass or shovel the snow?
- Can you repair broken items or change a light bulb?
- What would you do if you had a broken appliance?
- Do you do your laundry?
- Can you sew on a button?
- Do you clean your home?
- Who cooks at home?
- What do you use to cook with?
- Do you plan your menu?
- What do you usually eat for dinner?
- Who does dishes?
- How do you grocery shop (e.g., make list, drive to, use coupons, read newspaper ads, etc.)?
- How would you pay?

Financial Management
- Who pays your bills?
- Who balances your budget?
- Do you have trouble seeing $ or ✓s?

Leisure

- What do you do for fun?
- Are you interested in learning other leisure tasks?
- Are there any barriers that would interfere with your participation in leisure tasks?
- Are there groups you would like to be involved with or rejoin (church activities, bowling league, bridge club, etc.)?
- What are your favorite toys?
- Who do you play with?

Safety Procedures and Emergency Responses

- If you have a fire that you can't control, what do you do?
- If you cut yourself, what do you do?
- If you fall, what do you do?
- How will you get out of your house in an emergency?

Movement Function

Observe client's posture/mobility, the ability to stabilize and align him- or herself in relation to tasks for efficient use of UE. Functional observation of client when bathing, dressing, grooming, bending, and reaching using the following scale:

- *Good (WFL):* Able to sit/stand on flat surfaces without external or hand support
- *Modified Independence:* Client uses assistive device without supervision for balance while standing
- *Supervision (standby assist):* Needs supervision to maintain balance to ensure safety
- *Minimal Assistance (contact guard assist):* Therapist provides 25% or less support to maintain balance
- *Moderate Assistance:* Therapist provides 26%–50% support to maintain balance
- *Maximum Assistance:* Therapist provides 51%–75% support to maintain balance
- *Total Assistance:* Therapist provides greater than 75% support to maintain balance

Performance Tasks

- Place can on shelf
  - Note height of surface/type of surface (e.g., table)
  - Note if client is sitting or standing
- Retrieve item from floor
  - Use sock roll
  - Note if client is sitting or standing
- Screw lid on jar
  - Use peanut butter jar
  - Lid should be tightened to the point it is not loose (i.e., "snug")
  - Note if client holds jar on table, on lap, or in mid-air
  - Note which hand turns lid and how jar is stabilized
- Comb back of head
  - Client can be sitting or standing
  - Comb is held in right hand and transferred to left hand
- Write name
  - Client is seated with paper positioned on a comfortable height table in front of client with forearm resting on table
  - Client writes name with dominant hand; if unable because of motor deficits, non-dominant hand is attempted
- Lift a grocery bag (5 lb. bag of flour in bag)
  - Client may be sitting or standing
  - Note grasp pattern
  - Note approximately how high client can lift bag (e.g., knee height, waist height, table top, etc.)

Page 4—Cardinal Hill Healthcare System Protocol for Adult Occupational Therapy Evaluation, Short Form

Quality of Movement Scale/Evaluation Questions

Not functional

No attempt made with involved arm. No movement initiated. Neglects involved extremity. Involved arm does not participate functionally; uninvolved arm may be used to move the involved extremity.

Stabilizer

Requires assistance of uninvolved extremity for minor readjustments or change of position, or accomplishes very slowly. In bilateral tasks, the involved extremity serves as a helper or stabilizer.

Gross assist

Movement is influenced to some degree by synergy or is performed slowly and/or with effort. Primitive grasp patterns may be present. May need cues to integrate extremity during task performance. Uses involved limb to secure wheelchair lock with cues.

Functional

Movement is close to normal or appears to be normal; may be slightly slower or lack precision, fine coordination, or fluidity.

Use the following questions to aid in making comments and describing the client's movement during task performance. Not all questions will be applicable or necessary to describe the movements. Comment on only those questions applicable and most important to establish baseline and discharge data.

During task performance, does the client

- Have adequate muscle tone bilaterally to perform task? Does the tone fluctuate during task performance? Note the type and/or degree of muscle tone (e.g., severe hypertonia).

- Have adequate joint mobility (AROM and PROM) bilaterally to perform task? Note limitations in AROM and PROM of joints involved in movement to complete task. Use percentages (%) to describe range of movement (e.g., client has 50% AROM of shoulder flexion).

- Have adequate strength and effort bilaterally to perform the task? Assign muscle grade if necessary (e.g., 3+/5 for elbow extension). Comment on how client moves, transports, lifts, and calibrates objects.

- Have adequate muscle endurance to complete the task (e.g., do muscles tire before the task is completed?)?

- Have appropriate righting reactions, supporting reactions, eye–hand coordination, bilateral integration, and eye–foot coordination to complete the task?

- Present with substitution or synergistic movements while performing a task?

- Present with motor reflexes (e.g., ASTNR) or involuntary movements (e.g., tremors, tics, motor perserveration, associated reactions) during task performance?

- Use a specific grasp pattern or an abnormal grasp pattern? Comment on the type of grasp pattern used (e.g., hook grasp, cylindrical grasp, power grasp). If abnormal, describe the grasp.

- Use adaptive equipment to complete the task (e.g., reacher, adapted utensils)?

- Use upper extremity as a stabilizer, gross assist, etc. (refer to quality of movement scale for clarification)?

Energy for Task

Sustained effort over course of task performance

Within functional limits

Completes tasks without evidence of fatigue, rest break, or catching breath for 15 minutes or more, paces self, maintaining a consistent effective rate. Heart rate within 20 beats of resting rate and/or SpO_2 level above 95.

Fair

Demonstrates fatigue, minimal shortness of breath, need for rest break during dressing, grooming, chair transfers, reaching into cupboards, and moderate activity. Less than 15 minutes. SpO_2 level below 95.

Poor

Need for more than two rest breaks, moderate shortness of breath during 15 minutes or less of dressing, grooming, chair transfer, reaching into cupboards, moderate activity. SpO_2 level below 90.

Coordination

Note WFL or impaired. Further comment on gross motor, fine motor, eye–hand, eye–foot, and bilateral integration.

Hand Strength Tests

Grip Strength

"I want you to hold the handle like this and squeeze as hard as you can." Examiner demonstrates and then gives the dynamometer to subject. After subject is positioned appropriately, examiner says, "Are you ready? Squeeze as hard as you can." As client begins to squeeze, say "Harder! Harder! Relax." After the first trial score is recorded, the test is repeated with the same instructions for the second and third trial and for the other hand.

Tip (2 Point) Pinch

Tip Pinch is thumb tip to index finger tip. "I want you to place the tip of your index finger on this side as if to make an 'O.' Curl your other fingers into your palm as I'm doing."

Key (Lateral) Pinch

Key Pinch is thumb pad to lateral aspect of middle phalanx of index finger. "I want you to place your thumb on top and your index finger below as I'm doing and pinch as hard as you can." (Continue instructions as for Tip Pinch above.)

Palmer (3 Jaw Chuck) Pinch

Palmer Pinch is thumb pad to pads of index and middle fingers. "I want you to place your thumb on this side and your first two fingers on the side as I'm doing and pinch as hard as you can." (Continue instructions as for Tip Pinch above.)

Knowledge and Organization

Knowledge and Organization

- Choose, use, and handle tools (ADL equipment) and materials for intended purposes with good hygiene and in an appropriate manner, protecting objects from damage or dropping?
- Heed using goal-directed actions without "environmental" distractions?
- Seek verbal or written information without asking unnecessary information?
- Initiate tasks without hesitation, sequence tasks in logical order with efficiency, and terminate tasks appropriately?
- Gather needed and misplaced materials?
- Organize tools in logical positions of use?
- Restore tools by putting away and cleaning up?
- Navigate using UE, movement patterns to maneuver around objects without disturbance?

Note WFL or impaired and support with observations.

Adaptation/Praxis

Note WFL or impaired and support with observations; also describe any apraxias.
- Relate to the ability to anticipate, correct for, and benefit by learning from consequences of errors that arise in course of task performance.
- Notice/respond appropriately to nonverbal environment/perceptual cues (i.e., movement, sound, smells, and progress in task).
- Observe spatial arrangement of objects to one another, aligning objects as needed with effective/efficient response.
- Accommodate by modifying actions or location of objects in anticipation of problems that might arise.
  - Change method/sequence of task?
  - Change manner of tool use?
  - Ask for assistance when needed?
- Adjust—anticipate response to problems that might arise, making appropriate changes.
  - Move in space?
  - Use tools for intended purpose?
  - Turn off water?
  - Adjust temperature?
- Benefit—Anticipate and prevent undesirable circumstances from recurring or persisting.
  - Demonstrate home safety?

Observe client for indications of difficulty with completing task on command, or dressing skills, using the following descriptions and definitions. Can client follow basic commands during ADL task and evaluation, ruling out motor deficits?

Functional Observations
Difficulty with setting a table, making a sandwich, copying, drawing, and constructing two and three dimensions.

Further Test: Graphic
Copy geometric shape. Drawing without model (e.g., clock, house, flower).

Assembly
Three-dimensional block design.

Further Tests
Test of intransitive (express feelings) limb apraxia:
- Wave good-bye
- Beckon "come here"
- Finger on lip for "shh"
- Signal "stop"

Test of transitive (involve object use) limb apraxia:
- Brush teeth
- Shave face
- Hammer nail
- Saw board
- Use screwdriver

Social Interaction Skills

Comment on client's social interaction skills by using the following guidelines:
- Has client been able to go see family and friends or go out to dinner or shopping? Has he or she gone back to church or club activities?
- Does client need anger management or conflict resolution training for healthier coping skills?
- Can client express basic needs and wants? Does client express him-/herself in writing, orally, etc.? Can client identify basic ADL items?

Observation Skills
Does client make eye contact? Is he or she able to maintain a conversation? If client is aphasic, how does he or she interact: with nods, yes/no, communication board or u/a, depend on family member or caregiver? Does he or she pick up facial expressions (e.g., TBI u/a to pick up social cues)?

Auditory Skills
Does client have hearing aids, or is he or she hard of hearing in one or both ears? Does he or she use sign language? Is English his or her primary or secondary language?

Communication Device Use
- Is client able to use the phone, remote for TV?
- What does client do in an emergency (for D/C: lifeline device)?

Social Participation
- If client needed help, who would he or she call?
- Does client feel at this time he or she could socialize with friends, family, strangers?
- Does anxiety prevent client from participating in any occupations?

Cognitive, Affective

Level of Arousal
- Comment on ease of arousal during ADL.
- Note the amount of stimuli needed to arouse (stimulus—any sensory input including voice, touch, movement, cold, wet washcloth to the face).
- Note the time client is able to maintain arousal level without reintroducing stimulus.

Attention Functions
- How much cueing does client need to attend during initial evaluation or ADL/IADL task? Note the amount of time client can attend to the task. Can client attend to one task (note whether the environment is busy/noisy or calm/quiet)?

Page 7—Cardinal Hill Healthcare System Protocol for Adult Occupational Therapy Evaluation, Short Form

- Can client complete multiple-step tasks (note number of steps client is able to complete and again note the environmental context)?
- Comment on client's ability to attend during divided-attention tasks.

Orientation

- Can client perform routine/rote motor commands during basic ADL tasks? Can client perform non-routine/unfamiliar ADL tasks? Note how much cueing or modeling client requires to complete the task.
- If unable to assess at admission, write "to be assessed" on evaluation and complete during treatment while documenting in progress note.
- Can client take instructions learned during treatment and generalize them to ADL/IADL tasks? Is client realistic about injury/deficits and appropriate goals in rehab? Can client find unfamiliar rooms in hospital (e.g., gift shop, vending machine) for topographical orientation?
- Can client perform non-routine/unfamiliar ADL tasks? Note how much cueing or modeling client requires to complete the task. Can client perform check writing, money management tasks, medication regime, and meal planning (within dietary parameters)?

Emotional functions
Can client regulate emotions in response to task at hand? Can client control his or her emotions (e.g., is he/she labile)?

Self-esteem
Note client's confidence in ability to participate in ADLs and ability to regain functional ADL abilities. Does client make positive comments about self and abilities?

Sensory

Sensory Stimulation
- For each sensory stimulation item, comment on the following:

Type of Response
Note response as follows:
General Response (code GR): Client responds to stimuli in a non-specific way.
Example: Light touch to arm produces total body movement; noxious stimuli produces trunk extension.
Localized Response (code LR): Client responds to stimuli in a specific way.
Example: With light touch to arm, client pushes object away or moves arm; noxious stimuli produces head turn toward object or an effort to push object away.
No Response (code NR): Client exhibits no response to presented stimuli.

Response Rate
Indicate approximate percentage of response to stimuli when this information is important.

Comments
Indicate when/how responses were elicited and any other sensory stimulation information that would assist in understanding and treatment of client.

Tactile
- Comment on how client responds to touch and temperature of washcloth.

Further test:
Light Touch: Touch client's arm, trunk, or face with a feather, piece of fur, or paint brush.
Deep Pressure: Stimulate client's arm with deep pressure from therapist's hand.
Pain: Pinch nail beds on hand and feet for recognition of pain on both right and left side.
Temperature: Use ice or hot/cold test tubes to test both upper extremities.
- Does client respond to temperature of water when grooming, look to extremity being touched?

Further test:
Light Touch: Lightly touch client's skin with fingertip or paintbrush. Have client say "yes" or nod head each time stimulus is felt. For localization to touch, have client point to area touched.
Temperature: A tube of hot water and a tube of ice water are lightly placed on client's arm in a random manner. The client is to state hot or cold when he or she feels a stimulus. (Hot = 104°–113°; Cold = 41°–50°; dried off before presentation.)
Sharp/Dull: Give instructions to client. Begin the testing on an area of intact sensation, using point of safety pin for sharp and other end of safety pin for dull.
Semmes–Weinstein Monofilaments Test of Sensation: Start with monofilament number 2.83. Instruct client to hold out hands in supinated position side by side. Instruct client to respond to sensation by moving the finger that was touched. Obstruct client's vision. Touch the monofilament to each finger (test monofilament "breaks") and hold for 1 ½ seconds. Record the number of monofilament to which the client accurately responds including each finger/thumb. Indicate diminished sensation due to calluses. See key on evaluation form.

1.65–2.83 = WNL
3.22–3.61 = Diminished light touch
3.84–4.31 = Diminished protective sensation
4.56–6.45 = Loss of protective sensation
6.65   = Deep pressure sensation only

<u>Two-Point Discrimination:</u> The stimulus may be applied using a blunt-ended calibrated compass, Boley gauge, esthesiometer, or paper clip. The two points, separated by 2 mm, are applied along the longitudinal axis in the center of the zone to be tested. The two points are applied simultaneously and with equal, light pressure to the skin of the palmar surface of the palm and fingers. Heavy pressure invalidates the test by allowing the subject to perceive the two points when he or she would not be able to if correct pressure were used. One-point application trials are randomly interspersed with two points at 2 mm; the separation between the two points is increased by 1mm.

Proprioception

- Note client's response when upper extremity, lower extremity, and trunk are positioned. Does client position arms to brush hair or teeth? Does client know arm is off lapboard or is client aware of laying on hemi-arm?

- One extremity is positioned by the evaluator, and client is asked to match the position with his or her other extremity; vision is occluded; one or more joints may be involved in the tested position.

- Also considered in proprioception testing can be the accuracy of client's pointing response in the previous vision-occluded sensory tests.

Auditory

- Comment on how client responds to name, localization to sound.

Further test:
<u>Response to Voice:</u> Note how client responds when name called throughout session; speak from left and right side of client.
<u>Response to Music:</u> Note how client responds to a variety of music types.
<u>Noxious Noises:</u> These may include loud hand clapping, rattling a jar of beans, ringing a bell—present from left and right.

Vestibular

- Comment on how client responds when rolling, side-lying to sit, etc.

Further test:
<u>Fast/Slow:</u> Describe how client responds to different speeds of rolling, rocking.
<u>Rock/Bounce:</u> Describe how client responds to rocking, bouncing when in supine or sitting position.

Gustatory

- Comment on how client responds to a variety of solids and liquids, to oral care—by opening mouth or munching. Any hypersensitivities?

Further test:
Use a cotton swab to present the following stimuli to the client's mouth:
<u>Pleasant:</u> Fruit flavors
<u>Noxious:</u> Vinegar, peppermint

Olfactory

- Comment on whether client responds to smell of deodorant soap, aftershave, or perfume with increased movement or localized response.

Further test:
Note client's response to these types of stimuli presented in a small container or test tube and moved underneath client's nose.
<u>Pleasant:</u> Perfume, vanilla, fruit scents, etc.
<u>Noxious:</u> Ammonia, vinegar, etc.
Stimuli is presented for 1 second. Unaffected extremity should be evaluated first for a brief assessment. When testing dermatomes, see Spinal Cord Sensory Addendum (Appendix J). If client does not want to close his/her eyes, use a blindfold to occlude client's vision.
I = Intact, consistently able to respond correctly.
Mild = A few inconsistent or delayed responses are noted.
Moderate = 50% of responses are inconsistent, inaccurate, or delayed.
Severe = 75% of responses are inconsistent, inaccurate, or delayed.
Absent = Client is unable to feel stimulus.
Unable = Client is unable to participate or understand instructions in order to give an accurate response.

Visual

- Recommend a vision screen for all neurological clients. If deficits present, evaluate further following this key.

- Comment on how client watches you when walking around the bed or talking about ADLs.

Page 9—Cardinal Hill Healthcare System Protocol for Adult Occupational Therapy Evaluation, Short Form

Further test: None

Sudden Visual Stimuli: Note how client responds to object suddenly placed in field of vision.

Light/Dark: Note how client responds to suddenly turning on/off lights.

Familiar Picture: Note how client responds to a familiar picture placed in field of vision.

Acuity

• Does client, without trouble, recognize faces? Is print fuzzy or blurry, etc.?

Further test:

Near: Place Snellon Vision Card 14" from client's eyes. Client reads largest line first, moving downward. Examiner notes smallest line client can read in entirety or the line in which fewer than half the letters are missed. Record that the client has difficulty reading small print if 20/100 or less.

Far: Client stands/sits 20' from chart and reads rows of letters down the chart. Scoring is the same as Snellon Near testing above.

Oculomotor Control

• Does client complain of double vision? Does he or she squint, blink excessively, resist head change, etc.?

Further test:

Ocular Pursuits/Tracking

The client is asked to track a moving object to assess quality of eye movement. Examiner holds object 12"–16" from client's eyes, moving it slowly in vertical, horizontal, and diagonal patterns. Client is instructed to "move just your eyes, not your head." Assess whether tracking ability can be done simultaneously with range-of-motion evaluation.

Rating scale:

Intact: Client moves eyes smoothly with no jerkiness, able to maintain fixation, with no head movement.

Impaired: Eye movement is not smooth, client is unable to maintain fixation on object on one or both sides, client is unable to isolate head from eye movement, eye movement is slower to the involved side.

Convergence/Divergence

Medial and lateral rotation of eyes, which causes the lines of vision of the two eyes to meet on the target. Hold a bright object approximately 18" away from client's eyes; slowly move inward toward eyes, noting medial rotation of eyes. The closest point the client can fixate on target with both eyes is the convergence near point (CNP).

Rating scale:

Intact: Smooth, symmetrical medial rotation of both eyes up to approximately 9"–12".

Impaired: Asymmetrical movement of one or both eyes, CNP >12".

Saccades

Two brightly colored objects are held 12"–18" from client's eyes, approximately 12" apart. Client is asked to look back and forth, from one object to the other, on demand. Examiner then changes the position of the objects as client attends to the opposite object.

Rating scale:

Intact: Rapid, smooth, localization/fixation on target (slight under- or overshooting is normal).

Impaired: Under- or overshooting; long delay in fixating on object (>1 second); inability to isolate head and eye movement; jerky eye movements.

Eye Alignment

If client complains of double vision despite adequate ROM, ocular alignment should be assessed further. Perceiving a single visual image is dependent on both eyes receiving an image of an object on the corresponding retinal area of each eye. If the visual image falls on the fovea of one eye but not the other, a double image may be perceived.

Corneal Reflection Test

In dimly lit room, a penlight is held vertically under client's nose, so as to shine a reflection into each eye. A reflection off cornea in each eye should be observed, symmetrically placed in each eye, relative to the pupil.

Rating Scale:

Intact: Symmetrical reflections relative to pupil in left and right eye.

Impaired: Asymmetrical reflections (e.g., one reflection in center of pupil, one to left of pupil).

Cover/Cross Cover Test

Client asked to fixate at examiner's nose, slightly lateral to midline. Without telling client in advance, quickly cover one of client's eyes with small card or paper (index card), moving it from chin upward in front of eye. Notice any movement of uncovered eye. Repeat on opposite eye.

Rating Scale:

Intact: No movement of uncovered eye.

Impaired: Uncovered eye moves to fixate on object.

Visual Fields

Does client start to one side, stay close to a wall when navigating, brush one side of head or teeth, etc.?

Quantity of Vision

When eyes are in straightforward position, normal visual fields are approximately 64° upward, approximately 75° downward, approximately 60° inward, and approximately 90° outward. Total visual field is approximately 80° wide. Perimeter testing is available through an ophthalmologist and should often be pursued. However, informal visual field testing can be completed in the following manner:

Confrontation: Examiner stands behind client and a second person sits directly in front of client. Client is asked to focus on a target 12"–18" from the client's eyes (could be examiner's nose). The examiner moves a dowel with a white tip from outside the visual fields toward midline (from the left, right, superior, and inferior positions). At least 10–15 passes of dowel are generally necessary to obtain adequate information about visual fields. Examiner notes deviations from standards listed above.

Rating Scale

Intact: Client's visual fields correspond with examiner's (assuming examiner's are normal) or are within 30% of visual fields listed above.

Impaired: Client's visual fields are at least 30% less than examiner's (assuming examiner's are normal) or norms listed above.

Attention/Scanning

Visual scanning is a motor activity driven by attention, both attention and scanning occurring simultaneously. Normal visual scanning occurs in very organized and efficient ways.

Comment on client's ability to navigate on unit, locate grooming items at sink, etc.

Further test:

Intrapersonal Space—Within 20" of trunk

Scanning With Structured Array: Consider using letter cancellation task.

Place paper on table at client's midline. Ask client to cross out specified letter or symbol on paper. Examiner notes time needed to complete, pattern of scanning (as seen in the order of items crossed out), attention to detail throughout, symmetry in left and right performance. If client is unsuccessful, examiner provides strategy for success, such as using left-to-right scanning pattern, using hand to lead visual search, using anchor, etc. Examiner notes client's success with adaptive strategy.

Rating scale:

Intact: Client uses organized, structured approach (e.g., left to right, top to bottom) and misses no details on left or right, within reasonable time.

Impaired: Client omits characters and uses a random, disorganized approach to scanning. Note client's ability to use compensatory strategies. Clients with visual field loss without an attention and/or scanning deficit may take up to 7 minutes to complete cancellation task but are able to use organized strategies and scanning patterns to do so.

Scanning With Unstructured Array

Line Bisection Test: Client is asked to mark the center point on each of the horizontal lines on the page.

Rating scale:

Intact: If Line Bisection Test used, client should be able to mark center of horizontal lines within 1 cm.

Impaired: In Line Bisection Test, client unable to mark center of lines within 1". Client unable to attend to detail.

Homonymous Hemianopsia

Blindness of right-sided or left-sided vision of both eyes.

Testing: The therapist sits facing the client. The individualized colored blocks are randomly placed (a minimum of two to each side) on the client's shoulder. Instructions are given: "You are allowed to turn your head. What color do you see?" (If aphasic, have client identify colors placed in front of him/her.) The client then responds verballly.

Color-Blind

Absence of or defect in the perception of colors. The most common class of color-blindness is based on the perception of red, green, and blue (termed the 1st, 2nd, and 3rd color factors, respectively). Color-blindness in which all colors are perceived as gray is termed *monochromasia*.

Glasses: Comment if client has glasses or not.

Perception

Body Image

Note client's ability to perform task with awareness of body scheme and R/L discriminate. Note amount of physical cueing and/or verbal cueing needed to attend to affected body parts. Note awareness client has of deficits in body scheme and body image. Does the client follow body commands during ADLs? Does client follow body part commands in ADLs?

Self-concept

Can client identify strengths and weaknesses about him-/herself? Does the client put self down frequently or make "I" statements? Does client appear inflexible or resistant to trying adaptive technique? Does client appear demanding of the therapist to assist in ADLs in a certain manner? Does client appear positive and confident in his/her ability to regain skills in the future?

Experience of Self and Time Functions

Is client aware of all body parts (note _____, etc.)? Does client display appropriate self-concept; is he/she aware of change since the injury? Does client make appropriate positive comments about self, or does he/she make inappropriate negative comments?

Figure Ground

Observe if client can complete the following:

- Can client find towel and/or washcloth on bed (same color)?

- Can client find ADL items located at sink?

- Can client find eyeglasses, etc., in cluttered drawer?

- Does client have trouble finding the sleeve of unicolor shirt, Frosting Position in Space?

- Can client find wheelchair lock?

  Test: In drawer, client points to four grooming items (e.g., comb, deodorant, toothpaste, toothbrush, towel, washcloth)
  Scoring:
  Intact: Client points to 4 items within 10 seconds per item.
  Impaired: Client points to 0–3 items or response is greater than 10 seconds
  Further test: MVPT, VOSP

Depth Perception

Observe if client can complete the following:

- Put toothpaste on toothbrush.

- Pour water into glass; position wheelchair for transfer.

- Put glasses on.

- Put washcloth in water stream.

- Position wheelchair for transfer.

  Scoring:
  Intact: Client correctly completed 2 of the examples.
  Impaired: Client responds correctly 0–1 times or response is greater than 10 seconds
  Further Test: None

Pain

Note client's painful reactions with movement; observe for facial grimaces, withdrawals. Ask client if he/she presently has pain and location of pain. Have client describe sensation of pain (e.g., dull, stabbing). Have client rate pain on 1–10 scale, 1 being lowest and 10 being highest.

Skin Integrity

- Bleeding, depth, drainage, exposed anatomical structures location, odor, pigment, shape, size, staging, progression, tunneling

- Digital and grid measurements, grading of sores, observations, palpations, photographic assessments, wound tracing

- Signs of infection

- Wound scar tissue: banding, pliability, sensation, and texture scar rating scales

- Note activities, positioning, and postures that aggravate the wound or scar or that produce or relieve trauma

Associated Skin

- Blistering, continuity of skin color, dermatitis, hair growth, mobility, temperature, texture, turgor

- *Note:* Assistive, adaptive, orthotic, protective, supportive, or prosthetic devices and equipment that may produce or relieve trauma to the skin

- *Note:* General observations

Note edema if hand size appears unequal. If appears equal, record "no significant edema noted," or if edema control is a goal, objective measure should be recorded using a volumeter or circumferential measure.

Hand Volumeter
Set to measure hand and distal forearm edema. Fill the volumeter tank to the highest level/slight overflow. Place the overflow receiving pail under the volumeter immersion. Instruct the client to immerse one hand into the volumeter tank with fingers three and four (long finger and ring finger) straddling horizontal bar near base of tank. Note measurements by transferring displaced water from pan into the 500 ml graduated cylinder. Note precise measurement in cylinder. Note edema by comparing amount of water displaced by each hand/distal forearm measurement.

Circumferential Measurements
Use plastic tape with respect to anatomical landmarks. Accuracy and reliability depend on consistency of tape placement and tension applied when pulling tape.
Guidelines: 10 cm. Up/down from lateral epicondyle, over, ulnar styloid, MCP, DIP, PIP, dorsal of hand.

Comments

Experience of Self and Time Functions
Does the client display any inappropriate motor behaviors in response to psychological events? Does the client act out physically during event, or is client able to control motor use in relation to event?

Emotional Functions
Can client regulate emotions in response to task at hand? Can client control emotions (e.g., is he or she labile)?

Sleep
Note client's routine sleep cycle prior and after injury/insult. Is client's sleep pattern quality or not? Does client have day/night reversed?

Temperament/Personality Functions
What was client's temperament or personality prior to injury? Note changes in personality post-injury. How does client's emotional state impact ADL/IADL participation?

Mental Functions at Language
Can client follow basic commands during ADL task and evaluation, ruling out motor deficits? Can client express basic needs and wants? Does client express him-/herself in written or oral format? Can client identify basic ADL items?

Cardiovascular and Respiratory Functions

- What meds are you on?

- Have you had heart surgery or high blood pressure?

- Do you have trouble breathing especially when bathing, dressing, or going up steps?

RPD = Rate of perceived dyspnea (How does client rate the difficulty with breathing while performing activities, ADLs, and IADLs; also known as Borg Scale 0–10)
$SO_2 = > 95\%$
If $SO_2 = < 90\%$, have client sit and PLB (pursed lip breathing)
DB = Diaphragmatic breathing
0 = Nothing at all
0.5 = Very, very slight (just noticeable)
1 = Very slight
2 = Slight
3 = Moderate
4 = Somewhat severe
5 = Severe
6 = More severe
7 = Very severe (must rest)
8 =
9 = Very, very severe
10 = Maximal (must stop activity)
Cardiac Protocol Formula
Max HR = 220 – age
0.5 to 0.75 (max HR – RHR) + RHR

Risks that interfere with participation of occupation
Initial (eval) (protocol)

- How do risks interfere with participation?

- How do the client's performance areas, skills, patterns, context, activity demands, and client factors interfere with his or her ability to participate in occupation? Base your report on client's goals and priorities based on the environment they will be living in.

How has occupational therapy facilitated participation in occupation in client's environment?
Discharge (eval) (protocol)

- How has occupational therapy facilitated participation in occupation in client's environment?

- How did client benefit from your treatment so that he or she may generalize what was learned to other environments (include home program, family teaching, adaptative equipment, assistive technology, and community resources that increase client's success)?

Equipment
Comment on equipment client had before admission, was provided during admission, and equipment that is being recommended.

ELOS
Comment on expected length of stay for client.

Goals Met
Identify which goals from treatment plan the client met during admission.

Goals Not Met
Identify which goals from treatment plan the client did not meet and why.

Number of Visits
For COS indicate the number of times the client attended therapy.

Reason for Discharge
Indicate reason for client discharge.

Discharge Recommendations/Referrals
Indicate the recommendations for client upon discharge and where the client was referred.

Therapist Signature and Date
Therapist must sign evaluation and put date completed.

Note. WFL = within functional limits; w/c = wheelchair; AROM = active range of motion; PROM = passive range of motion; ASTNR = asymmetrical tonic neck reflex; ADLs = activities of daily living; TBI = traumatic brain injury; u/a = unable; D/C = discharge; IADLs = instrumental activities of daily living.

Cardinal Hill Healthcare System Protocol for Pediatric Occupational Therapy Evaluation, Long Form

Cardinal Hill Healthcare System
Protocol for Pediatric Occupational Therapy Evaluation,
Long Form

Occupational Profile

An occupational profile is defined as information that describes the client's occupational history and experiences, patterns of daily living, interests, values, and needs.

1. **Client lives with** _____ **in** _____ **(e.g., house, trailer, apartment).**

   Who is the client (e.g., individual, caregiver, group, population)? Collects information for determining client's roles (e.g., sibling). Determines *physical context* (i.e., nonhuman aspects of contexts). Includes the accessibility to and performance within environments having natural terrain, plants, animals, buildings, furniture, objects, tools, or devices (AOTA, 2002, p. 613).

   EVALUATION QUESTIONS

   • How many people besides yourself live in your home?

   • Do you live in a house, trailer, or apartment?

2. **A typical day consists of: wake-up time_____ (a.m., p.m.); volunteer; work; bedtime _____(a.m., p.m.).**

   Temporal Context
   Location of occupational performance in time (e.g., stages of life, time of day, time of year, duration; AOTA, 2002, p. 613)

   Habits
   • Useful Habits: Habits that support performance in daily life and contribute to life satisfaction. Habits that support ability to follow rhythms of daily life.
   • Impoverished Habits: Habits that are not established. Habits that need practice to improve.
   • Dominating Habits: Habits that are so demanding they interfere with daily life. Habits that satisfy a compulsive need for order.

   Routines
   Occupations with established sequences (Christiansen & Baum, 1997, p. 6).

   Roles
   A set of behaviors that have some socially agreed upon function and for which there is an accepted code of norms (Christiansen & Baum, 1997, p. 603).
   • Care of Others (including selecting and supervising caregivers): Arranging, supervising, or providing care for others.
   • Care of Pets: Arranging, supervising, or providing care for pets and service animals.
   • Education: Includes activities needed for being a student and participating in a learning environment.
   • Formal Educational Participation: Including the categories of academic (e.g., math, reading, working on a degree), nonacademic (e.g., recess, lunchroom, hallway), extracurricular (e.g., sports, band, cheerleading, dances), and vocational (e.g., pre-vocational and vocational) participation.
   • Exploration of Informal Personal Educational Needs or Interests (Beyond Formal Education): Identifying topics and methods for obtaining topic-related information or skills.
   • Informal Personal Education Participation: Participating in classes, programs, and activities that provide instruction/training in identified areas of interest.
   • Work: Includes activities needed for engaging in remunerative employment or volunteer activities (Mosey, 1996, p. 341).
   • Employment Interests and Pursuits: Identifying and selecting work opportunities based on personal assets, limitations, likes, and dislikes related to work (Mosey, 1996, p. 342).
   • Employment Seeking and Acquisition: Identifying job opportunities, completing, and submitting appropriate application materials, preparing for interviews, participating in interviews and following up afterward, discussing job benefits, and finalizing negotiations.
   • Job Performance: Including work habits (e.g., attendance, punctuality, appropriate relationships with coworkers and supervisors, completion of assigned work, and compliance with the norms of the work setting; Mosey, 1996, p. 342).
   • Volunteer Exploration: Determining community causes, organizations, or opportunities for unpaid work in relationship to personal skills, interests, location, and time available.

   Habits, Routines, and Roles

   EVALUATION QUESTIONS

   • Can you walk me through a normal day, starting with the time you get up until you go to bed at night?

   • What level of education did you complete? Can you read and write?

   • How many days of the week do you follow this schedule? (Gives insight as to social patterns with community, family, peers.)

<u>Care of Pets:</u>

EVALUATION QUESTIONS

- Do you have pets? Who cares for your pets? What do you do if they're sick? Do you buy food, etc.? Do you walk your pets?

<u>Education:</u>

EVALUATION QUESTIONS

- Are you a student? What are your learning interests?

3. **What activities do you participate in for fun, and how often?**
   Reveals information such as cultural context (AOTA, 2002, p. 613).

   Cultural Context
   Customs, beliefs, activity patterns, behavior standards, and expectations accepted by the society of which the individual is a member. Includes political aspects, such as laws that affect access to resources and affirm personal rights. Also includes opportunities for education, employment, and economic support.
   Leisure and social participation will be addressed under the areas of occupation.

   Leisure
   "A nonobligatory activity that is intrinsically motivated and engaged in during discretionary time, that is, time not committed to obligatory occupations such as work, self-care, or sleep" (Parham & Fazio, 1997, p. 250).

   Social Participation
   Activities associated with organized patterns of behavior that are characteristic and expected of an individual or an individual interacting with others within a given social system (Mosey, 1996, p. 340).

4. **How do you learn best? (In rehab you will be learning new things; do you learn best by reading, watching a video, etc.?)**
   See protocol for IADLs for further explanation in the area of education.

5. **How familiar are you with technology?**
   Relates to the *virtual* and *personal contexts*.

   Virtual Context
   Environment in which communication occurs by means of airways or computers and an absence of physical contact.

   Personal Context
   "Features of the individual that are not part of a health condition or health status" (WHO, 2001, p. 17). Personal context includes age, gender, socioeconomic status, and educational status.

   EVALUATION QUESTIONS

   - Do you have/use a computer?
   - Do you need anything to help you use the computer?

6. **What motivates you to improve?**
   Relates to the *personal* and *spiritual* and *cultural contexts* according to the *Framework*.

   Spiritual Context
   The fundamental orientation of a person's life; that which inspires and motivates that individual.

   Cultural Context
   Refer to definition above.

   Personal Context
   Refer to definition above.

   EVALUATION QUESTIONS

   - Why did you choose to come here?
   - Why do you want to get better?

   You may also include this information in the client factor area under temperament and personality functions as well as energy and drive functions.

7. **How are you/your family coping with your current status?**

(Also refers to *spiritual* and *cultural contexts.*)

EVALUATION QUESTIONS

- How are you handling this?
- Are you anxious, depressed, positive?

Comment if client is labile, etc.

8. **Occupation List**

Initial: Identify 5 occupations you want/need to resume.

1._____

2._____

3._____

4._____

5._____

- May need to be completed after the analysis is completed and client has a good understanding of what occupational therapy is. The occupational therapist may help client with this section.
- This is a good time to redefine *occupational therapy.*
- This section drives the treatment plan and determines the goals for occupational therapy as determined by the client.

9. **At Discharge**

You can rate the outcome or discharge response in this section with a satisfied or unsatisfied response. If the client is cognitively able, you may want to use a 1–10 scale to get a more exact response.

Always consider the age-appropriate expectations for the child you are assessing when completing evaluation questions and observations.

Basic Activities of Daily Living (Basic ADLs)

Activities that are oriented toward taking care of one's own body (Rogers & Holm, 1994, pp. 181–202); also called personal activities of daily living (PADL).

Eating/Oral Motor

Eating

The ability to keep and manipulate food/fluid in the mouth and swallow it (O'Sullivan, 1995, p. 191; AOTA, 2000, p. 629).

Feeding

"The process of [setting up, arranging, and] bringing food [fluids] from the plate or cup to the mouth" (AOTA, 2000, p. 629; O'Sullivan, 1995, p. 191).

EVALUATION QUESTIONS OR OBSERVATIONS

- Does the child eat pureed/strained/ground/lumpy/cut-up, chunky/diced/all textures of food?
- Does the child demonstrate age-appropriate/no spillage/spillage when eating?
- Can the child finger feed him- or herself independently?
- Can the child scoop with a spoon and bring it to his or her mouth?
- Does the child use a spoon well or with poor/fair/good accuracy?
- Does the child use a fork well or with poor/fair/good accuracy?
- Does the child spill food/overstuff mouth/is a clean eater during feeding?
- Does the child use a knife to butter bread/cut soft foods?
- Does the child drink from a bottle/sippy cup/open cup?
- Can the child pour liquid from pitcher into cup with independence/supervision/assistance?
- Will the child eat only certain foods (limited diet)?

Grooming

Obtaining and using supplies; washing, drying, combing, styling, and brushing hair; caring for nails (hands and feet); caring for skin, ears, eyes, and nose; applying deodorant; cleaning mouth; brushing and flossing teeth.

EVALUATION QUESTIONS

- Does the child hold toothbrush independently/with assistance?
- Does the child brush teeth thoroughly/not thoroughly?
- Does the child exhibit acceptance/decreased acceptance of toothbrushing?
- Does the child prepare toothbrush with toothpaste independently/with supervision/with assistance?
- Does the child brush hair independently/with assistance?
- Does the child brush hair thoroughly/not thoroughly?
- Does the child exhibit acceptance/decreased acceptance of hair brushing?
- Does the child manage tangled hair independently/with assistance?
- Does the child allow/not allow nose to be wiped?
- Does the child wipe/blow nose independently/on request/with assistance?

Bathing/Transfer

Bathing

Obtaining and using supplies; soaping, rinsing, and drying body parts; maintaining bathing position; and transferring to and from bathing positions.

Tub transfers

Tub transfers include getting into and out of a tub or shower.

EVALUATION QUESTIONS

- Does the child demonstrate increased/decreased acceptance for bath/shower/hairwashing?
- Does the child wash face independently/with assistance?
- Does the child wash and dry body independently/with assistance from bath/shower?
- Does the child wash hands thoroughly/not thoroughly; independently/with assistance?
- Does the child sit in the tub independently/with assistance/using equipment?
- Does the child step in/climb in/scoot in tub independently/with assistance?

Dressing Upper Body/Dressing Lower Body

Selecting clothing and accessories appropriate to time of day, weather, and occasion; obtaining clothing from storage area; dressing and undressing in a sequential fashion; fastening and adjusting clothing and shoes.

EVALUATION QUESTIONS

- Does the child choose/need assistance to choose own clothing?
- Does the child don clothing independently/with minimum/moderate/maximum assistance?
- Does the child independently/with verbal cueing/with assistance turn clothing right side out?
- Does the child doff clothing independently/with minimum/moderate/maximum assistance?
- Is the child independent/dependent/progressing with shoe tying?
- How independent is the child with clothing fasteners (e.g., buttons, snaps, zippers, shoelaces)?

Toilet Training/Transfer

Toilet hygiene

Obtaining and using supplies; clothing management; maintaining toileting position; transferring to and from toileting position; cleaning body; and caring for menstrual and continence needs.

Toilet transfers

Toilet transfers include getting on and off the toilet.

EVALUATION QUESTIONS

- Is the child independent/dependent/progressing?
- Does the child follow imposed toilet training schedule/wear pull-ups/stay dry the majority of the time with occasional accidents/indicate diaper is soiled?
- Does the child manage clothing for toileting independently/with assistance?
- Does the child transfer onto potty chair/toilet independently/with assistance?

Problem Solving/Memory

Problem solving includes skills related to solving problems of daily living. This includes the initiation, sequencing, and self-correcting of tasks and activities.

EVALUATION QUESTIONS

- Does the child demonstrate difficulty with change in routine/request help when needed/request help with self-care tasks often/not know what to do if problems arise/demonstrate age-appropriate skills for ADL completion?

Sleep/Rest

A period of inactivity in which one may or may not suspend consciousness.

EVALUATION QUESTIONS

- Does the child sleep through the night soundly/sleep alone/sleep with parent?
- Does the child move frequently during sleep/demonstrate difficulty falling asleep?
- Does the child wake up frequently in the night?
- Is the child difficult/not difficult to wake in the morning?
- Does the child have night terrors/nightmares?
- What time does the child typically go to bed?
- What time does the child typically wake up?
- What time(s) does the child nap?
- How long does the child nap?

Other tests: HELP, Carolina Curriculum.

Instrumental Activities of Daily Living (ADL)

Activities that are oriented toward interacting with the environment and that are often complex and generally optional in nature (e.g., may be delegated to another; Rogers & Holm, 1994, pp. 181–202).

Community Mobility

Moving self in the community and using public or private transportation

EVALUATION QUESTIONS

- Does the child require parental supervision in community?
- Does the child need cues to recognize unsafe situations in the community?
- Does the child ride the bus to school independently/with aid?
- Does the child walk to school independently/with supervision/with assistance?
- Does the child cross the street safely/with assistance?
- Does the child ride a bike in neighborhood independently and safely (wear helmet)/with supervision/unable to ride a bike?
- Does the child use public transportation independently/with assistance?
- Does the child understand and use public signs independently/with assistance?

Home Management

Participation at home chores, snack/meal preparation, and knowing how to seek help or whom to contact.

EVALUATION QUESTIONS

- Is the child independent with household chores?
- Does the child require frequent reminders to complete chores?
- Is the child able/unable to get a simple snack?
- Is the child able/able with assistance/unable to open refrigerator door and obtain a drink?

Play

Any spontaneous or organized activity that provides enjoyment, entertainment, amusement, or diversion (Parham & Fazio, 1997, p. 252).

Play Exploration

Identifying appropriate play activities, which can include exploration play, practice play, pretend play, games with rules, constructive play, and symbolic play (Bergen, 1988, pp. 64–65).

EVALUATION QUESTIONS

- Does the child choose age-appropriate play choices?
- Does the child choose games/activities appropriate for a lower age level?
- Does the child participate in practice play/pretend play/games with rules/constructive play?
- Does the child demonstrate perseverance on certain activities/ability to explore new toys/activities?
- Does the child require encouragement/assistance to participate in new play acts?
- What are the child's favorite play choices?

Play Participation

Participating in play; maintaining a balance of play with other areas of occupation; and obtaining, using, and maintaining, toys, equipment, and supplies appropriately.

EVALUATION QUESTIONS

- Is the child able to play independently for _____ minutes/unable to play independently?
- Does the child participate in solitary play/parallel play/interactive play with peers and siblings?
- Does the child demonstrate appropriate/decreased frustration/tolerance during play.

Safety Procedures and Emergency Responses

Knowing and performing preventive procedures to maintain a safe environment as well as recognizing sudden, unexpected hazardous situations and initiating emergency action to reduce the threat to health and safety.

EVALUATION QUESTIONS

- Does the child take risks during play/demonstrate age-appropriate safety skills/act overly cautious during play?
- Does the child play roughly with peers?
- Is the child safe/unsafe in parking lot?
- Does the child run from his or her parent in the community?
- Does the child require constant supervision?
- Does the child cross the street safely/requires assistance?
- Is the child able/unable to use emergency phone numbers?

Comments

Further comments on IADLs.

Motor Skills (Movement Function)

Skills in moving and interacting with task, objects, and environment (A. Fisher, personal communication, July 9, 2001).

Supine Flexion Posture

Procedure
The child lies on the floor on his or her back. First, demonstrate the position and then ask the child to assume the position independently (e.g., "Now curl your head up and hold your legs up so you go into a ball and stay that way as long as you can"). Provide resistance to forehead and knees, saying "Don't let me push you."

Record
The number of seconds the child maintained the full flexion posture. Criteria for breaking posture are
1. Feet touching floor
2. Nape of the neck touching floor

Significance
Five-year-olds are expected to execute supine flexion position and hold it without resistance for a period of 11–20 seconds. Most 5-year-olds cannot maintain supine flexion with resistance (Bundy, Lane, & Murray 2002; Dunn, 1981).

Prone Extension Posture

Procedure
The child lies on the floor on his or her stomach. First, demonstrate the position, and then ask the child to assume the position independently ("Now bend your knees; lift your head, arms, chest, and legs off the floor and hold it").

Record
The number of seconds the child maintained total extension posture. Criteria for breaking the posture are
1. Knees resting on the floor
2. Arms or head or both coming to the floor.

Significance
Individuals age 6 years and older should be able to assume prone extension and hold it for 30 seconds (Bundy et al., 2002).

Sitting Posture/Balance
Relates to the stabilizing and aligning of one's body while moving in relation to task objects with which one must deal.

Stabilizes
Maintains trunk control and balance while interacting with task objects such that there is no evidence of transient (i.e., quickly passing) propping or loss of balance that affects task performance.

Aligns
Maintains an upright sitting or standing position, without evidence of a need to persistently prop during the task performance.

EVALUATION QUESTIONS AND OBSERVATIONS
- Does the child sit in upright position/slump in chair during desktop tasks?
- Does the child lean on elbows during sitting tasks?
- Does the child demonstrate posterior/anterior pelvic tilt during static/dynamic sitting tasks?
- Observe bilateral scapula in sitting, child walking on straight line, frequency of falls

Developmental Positions
Observe the following positions: supine, prone, four point, ring sitting, side sitting, tailor sitting, chair sitting, bench sitting.
Is the child able to attain/maintain position independently/with minimum assistance/moderate assistance/maximum assistance/is dependent for position?

Movement Function

Motor Reflex Functions
Stretch reflex, asymmetrical tonic neck reflex.

Involuntary Movement Reaction Functions
Righting reactions, supporting reactions.

Control of Voluntary Movement Functions
Eye–hand coordination, bilateral integration, eye–foot coordination.

Page 7—Cardinal Hill Healthcare System Protocol for Pediatric Occupational Therapy Evaluation, Long Form

Involuntary Movement Functions
Tremors, tics, motor preservation

Gait Pattern Functions
Walking patterns and impairments, such as asymmetric gait, stiff gait. (*Note:* Gait patterns are assessed in relation to how they affect ability to engage in occupations and in daily life activities.)

*See Outpatient Range of Motion & Strength Addendum to record measurements.

Reflexes
Automatic response to a given stimulus.
Observe reflexes such as ATNR, STNR, protective extension, etc., as appropriate for age. Record presence or absence of reflex and if appropriate or inappropriate for age.

Energy for Task

Energy
Refers to sustained effort over the course of task performance.

Endures
Persists and completes the task without obvious evidence of physical fatigue, pausing to rest, or stopping to catch one's breath.

Paces
Maintains a consistent and effective rate or tempo of performance throughout the steps of the entire task.

Attends
Maintains focused attention throughout the task such that the child is not distracted from the task by extraneous auditory or visual stimuli. Sustained effort over course of task performance.
Within functional limits: Completes tasks without evidence of fatigue, rest break, or catching breath for 15 minutes or more, paces self, maintaining a consistent effective rate. Heart rate within 20 beats of resting rate and/or SpO_2 level above 95.
Fair: Demonstrates fatigue, minimal shortness of breath, need for rest break during dressing, grooming, chair transfers, reaching into cupboards, and moderate activity of less than 15 minutes. SpO_2 level below 95.
Poor: Need for more than two rest breaks, moderate shortness of breath during 15 minutes or less of dressing, grooming, chair transfer, reaching into cupboards, moderate activity. SpO_2 level below 90.

Coordination

Relates to using more than one body part to interact with task objects in a manner that supports task performance.

Coordinates
Uses two or more body parts together to stabilize and manipulate task objects during bilateral motor tasks.

Manipulates
Uses dexterous grasp-and-release patterns, isolated finger movements, and coordinated in-hand manipulation patterns when interacting with task objects.

Flows
Uses smooth and fluid arm and hand movements when interacting with task objects.

EVALUATION QUESTIONS AND OBSERVATIONS
- Does child stick out tongue during tasks requiring a lot of effort?
- Does child clench or move one hand when performing a task with the other?
- Does child have difficulty weight shifting?
- Does child have difficulty with crossing the midline?
- Does child have difficulty with trunk rotation during reaching?
- Does child have difficulty pumping a swing?
- Does child have difficulty stabilizing paper when writing?
- Does child have difficulty doing hopscotch?
- Does child have difficulty hopping on one foot?

Visual Motor

Visual Motor Skills

The ability of the eyes and hands to work together on tasks such as writing.

EVALUATION QUESTIONS AND OBSERVATIONS

- What is the child's hand dominance?
- Is the pencil grasp mature/immature/emerging/inefficient, functional/modified, loose/tight?
- Is the pencil pressure light/heavy/appropriate?
- How does the child use the nondominant hand during writing: adequate/inadequate paper frequently slips during writing?
- What type of handwriting is used: printing/cursive/both printing and cursive?
- Is the child able/unable to print/use cursive for letters with/without visual reference?
- What is the quality of writing in regard to size of letters, alignment, spacing, reversals?
- What is the child's ability to copy from board: adequate/has difficulty?
- What is the child's ability to copy from dictation: adequate/has difficulty?

Adaptation/Praxis

Adaptation

Relates to the ability to anticipate, correct for, and benefit by learning from the consequences of errors that arise in the course of task performance.

Notices/responds:

Responds appropriately to (a) nonverbal environmental/perceptual cues (i.e., movement, sound, smell, heat, moisture, texture, shape, consistency) that provide feedback with respect to task progression and (b) the spatial arrangement of objects to one another (e.g., aligning objects during stacking). Notices and, when indicated, makes an effective and efficient response.

Accommodates:

Modifies his or her actions or the location of objects within the workspace in anticipation of or in response to problems that might arise. The client anticipates or responds to problems effectively by (a) changing the method with which he or she is performing an action sequence, (b) changing the manner in which he or she interacts with or handles tools and materials already in the workspace, and (c) asking for assistance when appropriate or needed.

Adjusts:

Changes working environments in anticipation of or in response to problems that might arise. The client anticipates or responds to problems effectively by making some change (a) between working environments by moving to a new workspace or bringing in or removing tools and materials from the present workspace or (b) in an environmental condition (e.g., turning the tap on or off, turning the thermostat up or down).

Benefits:

Anticipates and prevents undesirable circumstances or problems from recurring or persisiting.

Praxis

The ability of the brain to conceive of, organize, and carry out a sequence of unfamiliar actions (Ayres, 1979).

Components of praxis include rhythm, sequencing, ideation, motor planning, bilateral coordination, projected action sequences, execution/feedback, and organization of behavior/problem solving (May-Benson, 2005).

EVALUATION QUESTIONS AND OBSERVATIONS

- Does child demonstrate poor control and quality of movements?
- Does child have difficulty with force discrimination (e.g., flings object too hard)?
- Does child have difficulty climbing on/off equipment?
- Does child have difficulty approaching and kicking a ball?
- Does child have difficulty/resist repeating a sequencing of tasks more than 1–2X?
- Does child use only a restricted repertoire of play themes?
- Does child have difficulty with sequencing components of functional tasks like dressing or tying shoes?
- Does child have difficulty organizing a daily schedule?
- Does child have difficulty with imitation of movement sequences (e.g., diadochokinesis, thumb to finger touching, jumping jacks, skipping)?
- Does child have difficulty constructing (e.g., setting up complex towers with blocks)?
- Does child drop objects on floor and forget about them?
- Does child know what actions to use with a new toy?

- Does child often use a toy in the same way?
- Does child have difficulty pretending?
- Does child have difficulty identifying different solutions to a problem (e.g., different ways to ride a scooter)?
- Does child often say "I can't do it" or ask for help before attempting to solve a problem?
- Record quality of movement with different activities client demonstrated:

Regular/irregular
Coordinated/uncoordinated
Overshooting/undershooting
Accurate/inaccurate
Fluent/decreased fluency
Smooth/stiff
Perseveres through task/easily frustrated

Motor Test Grids
[Insert any standardized/norm-referenced test material here.]

Social Interaction Skills

Refers to conveying intentions and needs and coordinating social behavior to act together with people (Forsyth & Kielhofner, 1999; Forsyth, Salamy, Simon, & Kielhofner, 1997; Kielhofner, 2002).

Communication Device Use
Using equipment or systems such as writing equipment, telephones, typewriters, computers, communication boards, call lights, emergency systems, Braille writers, telecommunication devices for deaf people, and augmentative communication systems to send and receive information.

Physicality
Pertains to using the physical body when communicating within an occupation.

Contacts
Makes physical contact with others.

Gazes
Uses eyes to communicate and interact with others.

Gestures
Uses movements of the body to indicate, demonstrate, or add emphasis.

Maneuvers
Moves one's body in relation to others.

Orients
Directs one's body in relation to others and/or occupational forms.

Postures
Assumes physical positions.

Information Exchange
Refers to giving and receiving information within an occupation.

Articulates
Produces clear, understandable speech.

Asserts
Directly expresses desires, refusals, and requests.

Asks
Requests factual or personal information.

Engages
Initiates interactions.

Expresses
Displays affect/attitude.

Modulates
Uses volume and inflection in speech.

Shares
Gives out factual or personal information.

Speaks
Makes oneself understood through use of words, phrases, and sentences.

Sustains
Keeps up speech for appropriate duration.

Relations
Relates to maintaining appropriate relationships within an occupation.

Collaborates
Coordinates action with others toward a common end goal.

Conforms
Follows implicit and explicit social norms.

Focuses
Directs conversation and behavior to ongoing social action.

Relates
Assumes a manner of acting that tries to establish a rapport with others.

Respects
Accommodates to other people's reactions and requests.

Social Participation
Activities associated with organized patterns of behavior that are characteristic and expected of an individual or an individual interacting with others within a given social system (Mosey, 1996, p. 340).

Community
Activities that result in successful interaction at the community level (e.g., neighborhood, organizations, work, school).

Family
Activities that result in successful interaction in specific required and/or desired familial roles (Mosey, 1996, p. 340).

Peer, Friend
Activities at different levels of intimacy, including engaging in desired sexual activity.

EVALUATION QUESTIONS

- Does the child readily greet therapist/present as shy/fearful/respond to greeting with prompting from parent/does not respond to greeting?

- Does the child need anger management or conflict resolution training for healthier coping skills?

- Can client express basic needs and wants? Does the client express himself or herself verbally, through writing, etc.?

- *Observation Skills:* Does the client make eye contact? Is her or she able to maintain a conversation? For example, if the client has aphasia, how does he or she interact with others—with nods, yes/no, communication board or u/a, depends on family member or caregiver? Does he or she pick up facial expressions?

- *Auditory Skills:* Does the client have hearing aids, or is he or she hard of hearing in one or both ears? Does he or she use sign language? Is English the client's primary or secondary language?

- *Social Participation:*
  Does child demonstrate stranger anxiety in community?
  Does child demonstrate anxiety in social situations?
  Does child interact socially at age-appropriate level with peers/siblings?

Cognitive Perceptual & Affective

Thought Functions
Recognition, categorization, generalization, awareness of reality, logical/coherent thought, appropriate thought content.

Higher Level Cognition
Judgment, concept formation, time management, complex problem solving, decision making.

Mental Functions of Language
Able to receive language and express self through spoken and written or sign language. (*Note:* This function is assessed relative to its influence on the ability to engage in occupations and in daily life activities.)

Calculation Functions
Able to add or subtract. (*Note:* These functions are assessed relative to their influence on the ability to engage in occupations and in daily life activities [e.g., making change when shopping].)

EVALUATION QUESTIONS AND OBSERVATIONS
- Does child regulate emotions in response to task?
- Does child demonstrate confidence in his or her abilities?
- Does child follow verbal commands? Child follows _____-step directions. Does child maintain standardized procedures?
- Does child require visual modeling for tasks?
- Does child follow physical demonstration?
- Is child aware of errors?
- Does child self-correct errors?
- Does child demonstrate perseveration with tasks?
- Does child require increased time to respond to questions/demands?
- Does child explore his or her environment?
- Child can/cannot tell time.
- Child can/cannot count coins/currency.

Consciousness Functions
Level of arousal, level of consciousness.

Attention Functions
Sustained attention, divided attention.

EVALUATION QUESTIONS AND OBSERVATIONS
- Does child present as awake and alert/drowsy/agitated?
- Does child demonstrate increased/decreased arousal level?
- Does child demonstrate difficulty modulating arousal level during evaluation?
  (Note if during the evaluation, attention is well maintained/the client is able to participate in standardized testing.)
- Is child unable to attend/demonstrates decreased attention/is distractible/responds to redirection (verbal cues, physical cues)/requires breaks?

Energy and Drive

Motivation, impulse control, interests, values.

Motivation
Observation of ADLs or functional task that motivates client. Interview client or family members to determine motivating factors. Cooperation during therapies and completion of ADLs.

Impulse Control
During ADL evaluate client's ability to control impulses. Note amount of physical and/or verbal cueing used by client to control impulsive behaviors.

EVALUATION QUESTIONS AND OBSERVATIONS

- Does child require encouragement to participate in tasks?
- Is child motivated to participate in tasks?
- Does child demonstrate impulsive behaviors interfering with task completion?

Sensory

Ability to perceive sensory input.

From a sensory integrative perspective, learning occurs when a person receives accurate sensory information, processes it, and uses it to organize behaviors. When children receive inaccurate or unreliable sensory input, their ability to process the information and create appropriate responses is disrupted (Dunn, McIntosh, Miller, & Shyu, 1999).

Vestibular System
Gives people a sense of movement and helps maintain equilibrium to keep the body upright against gravity. The vestibular receptors are in the inner ear.

Proprioceptive System
Allows people to guide their movements in a coordinated manner. The proprioceptive receptors are in the joints and muscles and sense the force of the muscles' tension to indicate the position of the body in space.

Tactile System
Allows people to sense what is being felt through the tactile receptors in the skin. It can protect people from feeling pain and helps discriminate the fine qualities of what is being felt. The tactile system is important in the development of a person's body scheme/image and affects emotions as well as arousal level (how alert a person feels).

Auditory Receptors
Are in the ears and provide information about what a person hears.

Visual Receptors
Are in the eyes and provide information about what a person sees.

Oral Receptors
Are in the mouth and provide information about what a person eats and drinks.

EVALUATION QUESTIONS AND OBSERVATIONS

- What does the child seek out/accept? Hair brushing/toothbrushing/baths/haircuts/hair washing/walking on grass, sand, cement without shoes/getting hands messy/playground equipment (swings)/climbing/jumping/spinning/touch from others/hugs and kisses/inappropriate objects to chew on.
- What causes overreaction or distress? Hair brushing/toothbrushing/baths/haircuts/hair washing/walking on grass, sand, cement without shoes/getting hands messy/playground equipment (swings)/loud noises/certain foods.

Additional Sensory Tests: The Sensory Profile

Sensory Test Grid
[Insert any standardized or norm-referenced test results here.]

Perception

Visual Perception
Visual perception is the brain's ability to perceive visual stimuli and process that information to respond appropriately in daily situations.

EVALUATION QUESTIONS AND OBSERVATIONS

- Does child confuse/reverse letters and numbers (e.g., the letters "b" and "d")?
- Does child have difficulty finding objects in competing backgrounds (e.g., a messy room, toy in a junk drawer)?
- Does child have difficulty putting puzzles together?
- Does child have difficulty imitating a block design?

Page 13—Cardinal Hill Healthcare System Protocol for Pediatric Occupational Therapy Evaluation, Long Form

Visual Perception Test Grid
[Insert any standardized/norm-referenced tests results here.]

Additional Visual Perception Tests
The Gardner Test of Visual Perceptual Skills (TVPS) and the *The Motor Free Visual Perceptual Test (MVPT)*

Visual

Seeing Functions
Visual acuity, visual field functions.

EVALUATION QUESTIONS
Acuity
- When was child's last vision exam at optometrist or ophthalmologist?

- Does client, without trouble, recognize faces?

- Is print fuzzy or blurry?

- Is child able to see the board at school?

Oculomotor Control
- Does client complain of double vision?

- Does client squint, blink excessively, complain of headaches when reading?

Further Tests

Ocular Pursuits/Tracking
Client is asked to track a moving object to assess quality of eye movement. Examiner holds object 12"–16" from client's eyes, moving it slowly in vertical, horizontal, and diagonal patterns. Client is instructed to move just the eyes, not the head. Assess that tracking ability can be done simultaneously with range-of-motion evaluation.
Rating Scale:
- Intact: Client moves eyes smoothly, with no jerkiness, able to maintain fixation, with no head movement.

- Impaired: Eye movement is not smooth, client is unable to maintain fixation on object on one or both sides, client is unable to isolate head from eye movement, eye movement is slower to the involved side.

Convergence/Divergence
Medial and lateral rotation of eyes, which causes the lines of vision of the two eyes to meet on the target. Hold a bright object approximately 18" away from client's eyes; slowly move inward toward eyes, noting medial rotation of eyes. The closest point the client can fixate on target with both eyes is the convergence near point (CNP).
Rating Scale:
- Intact: Smooth, symmetrical medial rotation of both eyes up to approximately 9"–12".

- Impaired: Asymmetrical movement on one or both eyes, CNP > 12 inches.

Saccades
Two brightly colored objects are held 12"–18" from client's eyes, approximately 12" apart. Client is asked to look back and forth, from one object to the other, on demand. Examiner then changes the position of the objects, as client attends to the opposite object.
Rating Scale:
- Intact: Rapid, smooth, localization/fixation on target (slight under- or overshooting is normal).

- Impaired: Under- or overshooting; long delay in fixating on object (> 1 second); inability to isolate head and eye movement; jerky eye movements.

Other Tests
Maples Ocular Motor Test

Comments

Psychomotor Functions
Appropriate range and regulation of motor response to psychological events.

Emotional Functions
Appropriate range and regulation of emotions, self-control.

Page 14—Cardinal Hill Healthcare System Protocol for Pediatric Occupational Therapy Evaluation, Long Form

Experience of Self and Time Functions
Body image, self-concept, self-esteem.

Psychomotor Functions
Does the client display any inappropriate motor behaviors in response to psychological events? Does the client act out physically during event or is client able to control motor use in relation to event?

Emotional Functions
Can client regulate emotions in response to task at hand? Can client control his or her emotions?

Sleep
Note client's routine sleep cycle prior and after injury/insult. Is the client's sleep pattern quality? Does client have day/night reversed?

Temperament/Personality Functions
What was the client's temperament or personality prior to injury? Note changes in personality post-injury. How does client's emotional state affect ADL/IADL participation?

Mental Functions at Language
Can client follow basic commands during ADL task and evaluation, ruling out motor deficits? Can client express basic needs and wants? Does the client express him- or herself in written or oral format? Can client identify basic ADL items?

Other Areas to Consider From the *Framework*

[To be noted in comments as appropriate.]

Occupational therapists and occupational therapy assistants have knowledge of these body functions and understand broadly the interaction that occurs between these functions as it is related to supporting performance and engagement in occupations and activities targeted. Some therapists may specialize in evaluating and intervening with a specific function:

• Voice and speech functions

• Digestive, metabolic, and endocrine system function

• Digestive system function

• Metabolic system and endocrine functions

• Genitourinary and reproductive functions

• Urinary functions

• Genital and reproductive functions

• Structure of the nervous system

• The eye, ear, and related structures

• Structures of the cardiovascular, immunological, and respiratory systems

• Structures related to the digestive system

• Structure related to the genitourinary and reproductive systems

• Structures related to movement

• Skin and related structures

Risks That Interfere With Participation of Occupation
Initial (eval) (protocol)
How do risks interfere with participation?
How do the client's performance areas, skills, patterns, context, and activity demands interfere with his or her ability to participate in occupation? Base your report on the client's goals and priorities based on the environment he or she will be living in.

How Has Occupational Therapy Facilitated Participation in Occupation in the Client's Environment?
Discharge (eval) (protocol)
How has occupational therapy facilitated participation in occupation in the client's environment?
How did the client benefit from your treatment, so that he or she may generalize what was learned to other environments (include home program, family teaching, adaptative equipment, assistive technology, and community resources that increase client's success)?

Equipment
Comment on equipment client had before admission, provided during admission, and equipment that is being recommended.

Duration
Comment on expected length of stay for client.

Goals Met
Identify which goals from treatment plan the client met during therapy.

Goals Not Met
Identify which goals from treatment plan the client did not meet and why.

Number of Visits
Indicate the number of times the client attended therapy.

Reason for Discharge
Indicate reason for client discharge.

Patient/Family Education
Indicate home programs and family education provided during therapy.

Discharge Recommendations and Referrals
Indicate the recommendations for client upon discharge and where the client was referred.

Therapist Signature and Date
Therapist must sign evaluation and put date completed.

References

American Occupational Therapy Association. (2000). Specialized knowledge and skills for eating and feeding in occupational therapy practice. *American Journal of Occupational Therapy, 54,* 629–640.

American Occupational Therapy Association. (2002). Occupational therapy practice framework: Domain and process. *American Journal of Occupational Therapy, 56,* 609–639.

Ayres, J. (1979). *Sensory integration and the child.* Los Angeles: Western Psychological Services.

Bergen, D. (Ed.) (1988). *Play as a medium for learning and development: A handbook of theory and practice.* Portsmouth, NH: Heinemann Educational Books.

Bundy, A., Lane, S., & Murray, E. (2002). *Sensory integration theory and practice* (2nd ed.). Philadelphia: F. A. Davis.

Christiansen, C., & Baum, C. (1997). *Occupational therapy: Enabling performance and well-being* (2nd ed.). Thorofare, NJ: Slack.

Dunn, W. (1981). *A guide to testing clinical observations in kindergarteners.* Rockville, MD: American Occupational Therapy Association.

Dunn, W., McIntosh, D. N., Miller, L. J., & Shyu, V. (1999). *Sensory Profile.* San Antonio, TX: PsychCorp.

Forsyth, K., & Kielhofner, G. (1999). Validity of the assessment of communication and interaction skills. *British Journal of Occupational Therapy, 62,* 69–74.

Forsyth, K., Salamy, M., Simon, S., & Kielhofner, G. (1997). *Assessment of communication and interaction skills.* Chicago: University of Illinois, Model of Human Occupation Clearinghouse.

Kielhofner, G. (2002). Dimensions of doing. In G. Kielhofner (Ed.), *A model of human occupation: Theory and application* (3rd ed.). Philadelphia: Lippincott Williams & Wilkins.

May-Benson, T. (2005). *Clinical assessment and practical interventions for praxis: From ideation to execution.* Columbus, OH: Professional Development Programs.

Mosey, A. C. (1996). *Applied scientific inquiry in the health professions: An epistemological orientation* (2nd ed.). Bethesda, MD: American Occupational Therapy Association.

O'Sullivan, N. (1995). *Dysphagia care: Team approach with acute and long-term patients* (2nd ed.). Bollingbrook, IL: Sammons Preston.

Parham, L. D., & Fazio, L. S. (Eds.). (1997). *Play in occupational therapy for children.* St. Louis, MO: Mosby.

World Health Organization. (2001). *International classification of functioning, disability, and health (ICF).* Geneva, Switzerland: Author.

Note. ATNR = asymmetrical tonic neck reflex; STNR = symmetrical tonic neck reflex; u/a = unable.

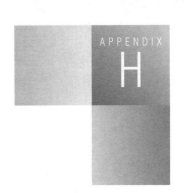

Cardinal Hill Healthcare System Occupational Profile (Pediatric)

Cardinal Hill Healthcare System
Occupational Profile (Pediatric)

Client Name: _____ Client #: _____ DOB: _____

Initial Date: _____ Discharge Date: _____

Diagnosis: _____

Precautions:_____

Occupational Profile:

1. Client lives with _____ in a house. _____
   _____

2. A typical day consists of: wake up time _____ ☐ a.m. ☐ p.m.; bedtime _____ ☐ a.m. ☐ p.m.
   _____
   _____
   _____
   _____
   _____

3. What activities do you participate in for fun and how often? _____
   _____

4. How do you learn best? (In rehab you will be learning new things. Do you learn best by reading, watching a video?) _____
   _____

5. How familiar are you with technology? _____

6. What motivates you to improve? _____

7. How are you/family coping with your current status? _____

Initial Comments   **Discharge Comments**

List 5 occupations you want/need to resume	Satisfaction in resuming your roles

_____ _____ _____ _____
Therapist's Signature   Date   Therapist's Signature   Date

Cardinal Hill
Healthcare System
Occupational Analysis
(Pediatric)

Cardinal Hill Healthcare System
Occupational Analysis (Pediatric)

Client Name: _____ Client #: _____ DOB: _____

Initial Date: _____ Discharge Date: _____

Diagnosis: _____ Precautions: _____

Age: _____ Grade in School: _____ Physician: _____

Occupational Analysis:

Initial Comments   **Discharge Comments**

	Basic ADLs	
	Eating/Oral Motor	
	Grooming	
	Bathing/Transfer	
	Dressing Upper Body	
	Dressing Lower Body	
	Toilet Training/Transfer	
	Problem Solving/Memory	
	Comments	

Age Equivalent	Percentile	Standard Score	ADL Test	Age Equivalent	Percentile	Standard Score

Note. This assessment form has been expanded to allow readers of all visual acuity to access its information. A 2-page form of this assessment can be found on the CD-ROM.

Page 1—Cardinal Hill Healthcare System Occupational Analysis (Pediatric)

Client Name: _____ Client #: _____

Initial Comments   **Discharge Comments**

	Instrumental ADLs	
	Community Mobility	
	Home Management	
	Play Exploration	
	Play Participation	
	Safety	
	Comments	
	Movement Function	
	Supine Flexion Posture	
	Prone Extension Posture	
	Sitting Posture/Balance	
	Developmental Positions	
	Muscle Functions	

Client Name: _____ Client #: _____

Initial Comments

	Movement Function	
	Reflexes	
	Comments	
	Energy for Task	
	Coordination	
	Manipulation	
	Visual Motor	
	Adaptation/Praxis	
	Comments	

Age Equivalent	Percentile	Standard Score	Motor Test	Age Equivalent	Percentile	Standard Score
Age Equivalent	Percentile	Standard Score	Motor Test	Age Equivalent	Percentile	Standard Score

Client Name: _____ Client #: _____

Initial Comments   **Discharge Comments**

	Social Interaction Skills	
	Cognitive Perceptual & Affective	
	Level of Arousal/Attention	
	Energy & Drive	
	Comments	

Sensory

Typical	Atypical	Sensory Test	Typical	Atypical

| | Comments | |

Perception

Age Equivalent	Percentile	Standard Score	Perception Test	Age Equivalent	Percentile	Standard Score

| | **Visual** | |
| | Comments | |

Page 4—Cardinal Hill Healthcare System Occupational Analysis (Pediatric)

Client Name: _____ Client #: _____

Initial Comments   **Discharge Comments**

How do the risks interfere with participation in occupation?	How has occupational therapy facilitated participation in occupation in client's environment?

Equipment: Equipment provided:

Duration: _____   Number of visits: _____

                                                 Reason for discharge: _____

                                                 Discharge goals met: _____

                                                 Discharge goals not met: _____

                                                 Patient/family education: _____

                                                 _____

                                                 _____

                                                 _____

                                                 Discharge recommendations/referrals: _____

                                                 _____

                                                 _____

                                                 _____

_____   _____   _____   _____
Therapist's Signature   Date   Therapist's Signature   Date

Page 5—Cardinal Hill Healthcare System Occupational Analysis (Pediatric)

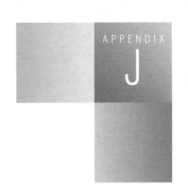

Cardinal Hill
Healthcare System
Range-of-Motion and
Sensation Addenda

Cardinal Hill Healthcare System Range-of-Motion Form

Client Name: _____   Client #: _____

Initial Comments				Range of Motion			Discharge Comments			
AROM		**PROM**					**AROM**		**PROM**	
L	R	L	R	Joint	Motion	ROM	L	R	L	R
				Shoulder	Flexion	180				
				Shoulder	Abduction	180				
				Shoulder	Int. Rotation	70				
				Shoulder	Ext. Rotation	90				
				Shoulder	Horiz. Abduction	90				
				Shoulder	Horiz. Adduction	45				
				Elbow	Flexion	135				
				Elbow	Extension	0				
				Forearm	Pronation	70				
				Forearm	Supination	80				
				Wrist	Flexion	75				
				Wrist	Extension	70				
				Wrist	Ulnar Deviation	30				
				Wrist	Radial Deviation	15				
				MCP 1	Flexion	90				
				MCP 2	Flexion	90				
				MCP 3	Flexion	90				
				MCP 4	Flexion	90				
				MCP 1	Extension	0				
				MCP 2	Extension	0				
				MCP 3	Extension	0				
				MCP 4	Extension	0				
				PIP 1	Flexion	100				
				PIP 2	Flexion	100				
				PIP 3	Flexion	100				
				PIP 4	Flexion	100				
				PIP 1	Extension	0				
				PIP 2	Extension	0				
				PIP 3	Extension	0				
				PIP 4	Extension	0				
				DIP 1	Flexion	90				
				DIP 2	Flexion	90				
				DIP 3	Flexion	90				
				DIP 4	Flexion	90				
				DIP 1	Extension	0				
				DIP 2	Extension	0				
				DIP 3	Extension	0				
				DIP 4	Extension	0				
				Thumb MP	Flexion	50				
				Thumb MP	Extension	0				
				Thumb IP	Flexion	80				
				Thumb IP	Extension	0				

Scapula: _____

Pain: _____

Edema: _____

Contracture: _____

Spasticity: _____

Splints Indicated: _____

Note. AROM = active range of motion; PROM = passive range of motion; Int = internal rotation; Ext = external rotation; Horiz = horizontal; MCP = metacarpal phalangeal joints; PIP = proximal interphalangeal joints; DIP = distal interphalangeal joints; MP = motor planning.

Page 1—Cardinal Hill Healthcare System Range-of-Motion Form

Cardinal Hill Healthcare System Sensation Form

Client Name: _____ Client #: _____

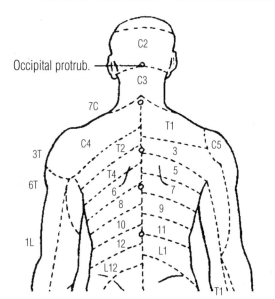

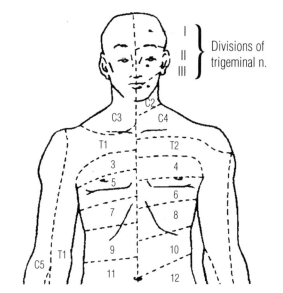

Sharp/Dull

	Right			Left		
	Int	Imp	Abs	Int	Imp	Abs
C3						
C4						
C5						
C6						
C7						
C8						
T1						
T2						

Position Sense

	Right			Left		
	Int	Imp	Abs	Int	Imp	Abs
Radial Fingers						
Ulnar Fingers						
Thumb						
Wrist						
Forearm Rot						
Elbow						
Shoulder						

Temperature

	Right			Left		
	Int	Imp	Abs	Int	Imp	Abs
C3						
C4						
C5						
C6						
C7						
C8						
T1						
T2						

Object Identification

	Right			Left		
	Int	Imp	Abs	Int	Imp	Abs

Light Touch

	Right			Left		
	Int	Imp	Abs	Int	Imp	Abs
C3						
C4						
C5						
C6						
C7						
C8						
T1						
T2						

Comments: _____

_____

_____

_____

_____

_____

Note. Int = internal rotation; Imp = impaired; Abs = absent.

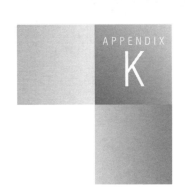

Occupational Therapy Practice Framework: Domain and Process

Occupational Therapy Practice Framework: Domain and Process

Contents

When citing this document the preferred reference is:

American Occupational Therapy Association. (2002). Occupational therapy practice framework: Domain and process. *American Journal of Occupational Therapy, 56,* 609–639.

Occupational therapy is an evolving profession. Over the years, the study of human occupation and its components has enlightened the profession about the core concepts and constructs that guide occupational therapy practice. In addition, occupational therapy's role and contributions to society have continued to evolve. The *Occupational Therapy Practice Framework: Domain and Process* (also referred to in this document as the Framework) is the next evolution in a series of documents that have been developed over the past several decades to outline language and constructs that describe the profession's focus.

The Framework was developed in response to current practice needs—the need to more clearly affirm and articulate occupational therapy's unique focus on occupation and daily life activities and the application of an intervention process that facilitates engagement in occupation to support participation in life. The impetus for the development of the Framework was the review process to update and revise the *Uniform Terminology for Occupational Therapy—Third Edition* (UT-III) (American Occupational Therapy Association [AOTA], 1994). The background for the development of the Framework is provided in a section at the end of this document. As practice continues to evolve, the field should consider the continued need for the *Occupational Therapy Practice Framework: Domain and Process* and should evaluate and modify its format as appropriate.

The intended purpose of the Framework is twofold: (a) to describe the domain that centers and grounds the profession's focus and actions and (b) to outline the process of occupational therapy evaluation and intervention that is dynamic and linked to the profession's focus on and use of occupation. The domain and process are necessarily interdependent, with the domain defining the area of human activity to which the process is applied.

This document is directed to both internal and external audiences. The internal professional audience—occupational therapists and occupational therapy assistants—can use the Framework to examine their current practice and to consider new applications in emerging practice areas. Occupational therapy educators may find the Framework helpful in teaching students about a process delivery model that is client centered and facilitates engagement in occupation to support participation in life. As occupational therapists and occupational therapy assistants move into new and expanded service arenas, the descriptions and terminology provided in the Framework can assist them in communicating the profession's unique focus on occupation and daily life activities to external audiences. External audiences can use the Framework to understand occupational therapy's emphasis on supporting function and performance in daily life activities and the many factors that influence performance (e.g., performance skills, performance patterns, context, activity demands, client factors) that are addressed during the intervention process. The description of the process will assist external audiences in understanding how occupational therapists and occupational therapy assistants apply their knowledge and skills in helping people attain and resume daily life activities that support function and health.

The *Occupational Therapy Practice Framework: Domain and Process* begins with an explanation of the profession's domain. Each aspect of the domain is fully described. An introduction to the occupational therapy process follows with key statements that highlight important points. Each section of the process is then specifically described. Numerous resource materials, including an appendix, a glossary, references, a bibliography, and the background of the development of the Framework are supplied at the end of the document.

Domain

The Domain of Occupational Therapy

"A profession's domain of concern consists of those areas of human experience in which practitioners of the profession offer assistance to others" (Mosey, 1981, p. 51). Occupational therapists and occupational therapy assistants focus on assisting people to engage in daily life activities that they find meaningful and purposeful. Occupational therapy's domain stems from the profession's interest in human beings' ability to engage in everyday life activities. The broad term that occupational therapists and assistants use to capture the breadth and meaning of "everyday life activity" is *occupation*. Occupation, as used in this document, is defined in the following way:

> [A]ctivities…of everyday life, named, organized, and given value and meaning by individuals and a culture. Occupation is everything people do to occupy themselves, including looking after themselves…enjoying life…and contributing to the social and economic fabric of their communities…. (Law, Polatajko, Baptiste, & Townsend, 1997, p. 32)

Occupational therapists' and occupational therapy assistants' expertise lies in their knowledge of occupation and how engaging in occupations can be used to affect human performance and the effects of disease and disability. When working with clients, occupational therapists and occupational therapy assistants direct their effort toward helping clients perform. Performance changes are directed to support engagement in meaningful occupations that subsequently affect health, well-being, and life satisfaction.

The profession views occupation as both means and end. The process of providing occupational therapy intervention may involve the therapeutic use of occupation as a "means" or method of changing performance. The "end" of

the occupational therapy intervention process occurs with the client's improved engagement in meaningful occupation.

Both terms, *occupation* and *activity*, are used by occupational therapists and occupational therapy assistants to describe participation in daily life pursuits. Occupations are generally viewed as activities having unique meaning and purpose in a person's life. Occupations are central to a person's identity and competence, and they influence how one spends time and makes decisions. The term *activity* describes a general class of human actions that is goal directed (Pierce, 2001). A person may participate in activities to achieve a goal, but these activities do not assume a place of central importance or meaning for the person. For example, many people participate in the activity of gardening, but not all of those individuals would describe gardening as an "occupation" that has central importance and meaning for them. Those who see gardening as an activity may report that gardening is a chore or task that must be done as part of home and yard maintenance but not one that they particularly enjoy doing or from which they derive significant personal satisfaction or fulfillment. Those who experience gardening as an occupation would see themselves as "gardeners," gaining part of their identity from their participation. They would achieve a sense of competence by their accomplishments in gardening and would report a sense of satisfaction and fulfillment as a result of engaging in this occupation. Occupational therapists and occupational therapy assistants value both occupation and activity and recognize their importance and influence on health and well-being. They believe that the two terms are closely related yet recognize that each term has a distinct meaning and that individuals experience each differently. In this document the two terms are often used together to acknowledge their relatedness yet recognize their different meanings.

The domain of occupational therapy frames the arena in which occupational therapy evaluations and interventions occur. To make the domain more understandable to readers and easier to visualize, the content of the domain has been illustrated in Figure 1. At the top of the page is the overarching statement—Engagement in Occupation to Support Participation in Context or Contexts. This statement describes the domain in its broadest sense. The other terms outlined in the figure identify the various aspects of the domain that occupational therapists and occupational therapy assistants attend to during the process of providing services. The three terms at the bottom of the figure (*context, activity demands,* and *client factors*) identify areas that influence performance skills and patterns. The two terms in the middle of the figure (*performance skills* and *performance patterns*) are used to describe the observed performance that

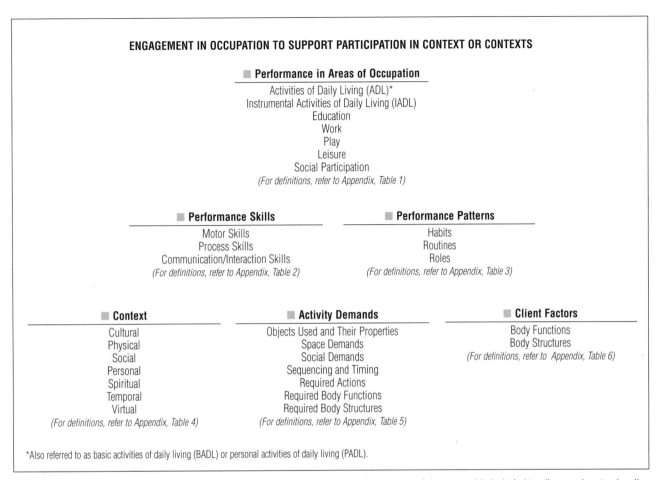

Figure 1. **Domain of Occupational Therapy.** This figure represents the domain of occupational therapy and is included to allow readers to visualize the entire domain with all of its various aspects. No aspect is intended to be perceived as more important than another.

the individual carries out when engaging in a range of occupations. No one aspect outlined in the domain figure is considered more important than another. Occupational therapists are trained to assess all aspects and to apply that knowledge to an intervention process that leads to engagement in occupations to support participation in context or contexts. Occupational therapy assistants participate in this process under the supervision of an occupational therapist. The discussion that follows provides a brief explanation of each term in the figure. Tables included in the appendix provide full lists and definitions of terms.

Engagement in Occupation to Support Participation in Context

Engagement in occupation to support participation in context is the focus and targeted end objective of occupational therapy intervention. Engagement in occupation is seen as naturally supporting and leading to participation in context.

When individuals engage in occupations, they are committed to performance as a result of self-choice, motivation, and meaning. The term expresses the profession's belief in the importance of valuing and considering the individual's desires, choices, and needs during the evaluation and intervention process. Engagement in occupation includes both the subjective (emotional or psychological) aspects of performance and the objective (physically observable) aspects of performance. Occupational therapists and occupational therapy assistants understand engagement from this dual and holistic perspective and address all the aspects of performance (physical, cognitive, psychosocial, and contextual) when providing interventions designed to support engagement in occupations and in daily life activities.

Occupational therapists and occupational therapy assistants recognize that health is supported and maintained when individuals are able to engage in occupations and in activities that allow desired or needed participation in home, school, workplace, and community life situations. Occupational therapists and occupational therapy assistants assist individuals to link their ability to perform daily life activities with meaningful patterns of engagement in occupations that allow participation in desired roles and life situations in home, school, workplace, and community. The World Health Organization (WHO), in its effort to broaden the understanding of the effects of disease and disability on health, has recognized that health can be affected by the inability to carry out activities and participate in life situations as well as by problems that exist with body structures and functions (WHO, 2001). Occupational therapy's focus on engagement in occupations to support participation complements WHO's perspective.

Occupational therapists and occupational therapy assistants recognize that engagement in occupation occurs in a variety of contexts (cultural, physical, social, personal, temporal, spiritual, virtual). They also recognize that the individual's experience and performance cannot be understood or addressed without understanding the many contexts in which occupations and daily life activities occur.

Performance in Areas of Occupation

Occupational therapists and occupational therapy assistants direct their expertise to the broad range of human occupations and activities that make up peoples' lives. When occupational therapists and assistants work with an individual, a group, or a population to promote engagement in occupations and in daily life activities, they take into account all of the many types of occupations in which any individual, group, or population might engage. These human activities are sorted into categories called "areas of occupation"—activities of daily living, instrumental activities of daily living, education, work, play, leisure, and social participation (see Appendix, Table 1). Occupational therapists and occupational therapy assistants under the supervision of an occupational therapist use their expertise to address performance issues in any or all areas that are affecting the person's ability to engage in occupations and in activities. Addressing performance issues in areas of occupation requires knowledge of what performance skills are needed and what performance patterns are used.

Performance Skills

Skills are small units of performance. They are features of what one does (e.g., bends, chooses, gazes), versus underlying capacities or body functions (e.g., joint mobility, motivation, visual acuity). "Skills are observable elements of action that have implicit functional purposes" (Fisher & Kielhofner, 1995, p. 113). For example, when observing a person writing out a check, you would notice skills of gripping and manipulating objects and initiating and sequencing the steps of the activity to complete the writing of the check.

Execution of a performance skill occurs when the performer, the context, and the demands of the activity come together in the performance of the activity. Each of these

factors influences the execution of a skill and may support or hinder actual skill execution.

When occupational therapists and occupational therapy assistants, who have established competency under the supervision of occupational therapists, analyze performance, they specifically identify the skills that are effective or ineffective during performance. They use skilled observations and selected assessments to evaluate the following skills:

- Motor skills—observed as the client moves and interacts with task objects and environments. Aspects of motor skill include posture, mobility, coordination, strength and effort, and energy. Examples of specific motor performance skills include stabilizing the body, bending, and manipulating objects.

- Process skills—observed as the client manages and modifies actions while completing a task. Aspects of process skill include energy, knowledge, temporal organization, organizing space and objects, and adaptation. Examples of specific process performance skills include maintaining attention to a task, choosing appropriate tools and materials for the task, logically organizing workspace, or accommodating the method of task completion in response to a problem.

- Communication/Interaction skills—observed as the client conveys his or her intentions and needs and coordinates social behavior to act together with people. Aspects of communication/interaction skills include physicality, information exchange, and relations. Examples of specific communication/interaction performance skills include gesturing to indicate intention, asking for information, expressing affect, or relating in a manner to establish rapport with others.

Skilled performance (i.e., effective execution of performance skills) depends on client factors (body functions, body structures), activity demands, and the context. However, the presence of underlying client factors (body functions and structures) does not inherently ensure the effective execution of performance skills. (See Appendix, Table 2, for complete list of performance skills)

Performance Patterns

Performance patterns refer to habits, routines, and roles that are adopted by an individual as he or she carries out occupations or daily life activities. Habits refer to specific, automatic behaviors, whereas routines are established sequences of occupations or activities that provide a structure for daily life. Roles are "a set of behaviors that have some socially agreed upon function and for which there is an accepted code of norms" (Christiansen & Baum, 1997, p. 603).

Performance patterns develop over time and are influenced by context (See Appendix, Table 3).

Context

Context refers to a variety of interrelated conditions within and surrounding the client that influence performance. These contexts can be cultural, physical, social, personal, spiritual, temporal, and virtual. Some contexts are external to the client (e.g., physical context, social context, virtual context); some are internal to the client (e.g., personal, spiritual); and some may have external features, with beliefs and values that have been internalized (e.g., cultural). Contexts may include time dimensions (e.g., within a temporal context, the time of day; within a personal context, one's age) and space dimensions (e.g., within a physical context, the size of room in which activity occurs). When the occupational therapist and occupational therapy assistant are attempting to understand performance skills and patterns, they consider the specific contexts that surround the performance of a particular occupation or activity. In this process, the therapist and assistant consider all the relevant contexts, keeping in mind that some of them may not be influencing the particular skills and patterns being addressed. (See Appendix, Table 4, for a description of the different kinds of contexts that occupational therapists and occupational therapy assistants consider.)

Activity Demands

The demands of the activity in which a person engages will affect skill and eventual success of performance. Occupational therapists and occupational therapy assistants apply their analysis skills to determine the demands that an activity will place on any performer and how those demands will influence skill execution. (See Appendix, Table 5, for complete list of activity demands.)

Client Factors

Performance can be influenced by factors that reside within the client. Occupational therapists and occupational therapy assistants are knowledgeable about the variety of physical, cognitive, and psychosocial client factors that influence development and performance and how illness, disease, and disability affect these factors. The occupational therapist and occupational therapy assistant recognize that client factors influence the ability to engage in occupations and that engagement in occupations can also influence client factors. They apply their understanding of this interaction and use it throughout the intervention process.

Client factors include the following:
- Body functions—"physiological function of body systems (including psychological functions)" (WHO, 2001, p. 10). (See Appendix, Table 6, for complete list.) The occupational therapist and occupational therapy assistant under the supervision of an occupational therapist use

knowledge about body functions to evaluate selected client body functions that may be affecting his or her ability to engage in desired occupations or activities.
- Body structures—"anatomical parts of the body such as organs, limbs, and their components" (WHO, 2001, p. 10). (See Appendix, Table 6.) Occupational therapists and occupational therapy assistants under the supervision of an occupational therapist apply their knowledge about body structures to determine which body structures are needed to carry out an occupation or activity.

The categorization of client factors outlined in Table 6 is based on the *International Classification of Functioning, Disability and Health* proposed by the WHO (2001). The classification was selected because it has received wide exposure and presents a common language that is understood by external audiences. The categories include all those areas that occupational therapists and assistants address and consider during evaluation and intervention.

Process
The Process of Occupational Therapy: Evaluation, Intervention, and Outcome

Many professions use the process of evaluating, intervening, and targeting intervention outcomes that is outlined in the Framework. However occupational therapy's focus on occupation throughout the process makes the profession's application and use of the process unique. The process of occupational therapy service delivery begins by evaluating the client's occupational needs, problems, and concerns. Understanding the client as an occupational human being for whom access and participation in meaningful and productive activities is central to health and well-being is a perspective that is unique to occupational therapy. Problems and concerns that are addressed in evaluation and intervention are also framed uniquely from an occupational perspective, are based on occupational therapy theories, and are defined as problems or risks in occupational performance. During intervention, the focus remains on occupation, and efforts are directed toward fostering improved engagement in occupations. A variety of therapeutic activities, including engagement in actual occupations and in daily life activities, are used in intervention.

Framework Process Organization

The *Occupational Therapy Practice Framework* process is organized into three broad sections that describe the process of service delivery. A brief overview of the process as it is applied within the profession's domain is outlined in Figure 2.

Figure 3 schematically illustrates how these sections are related to one another and how they revolve around the col-

■ **Evaluation**

Occupational profile—The initial step in the evaluation process that provides an understanding of the client's occupational history and experiences, patterns of daily living, interests, values, and needs. The client's problems and concerns about performing occupations and daily life activities are identified, and the client's priorities are determined.

Analysis of occupational performance—The step in the evaluation process during which the client's assets, problems, or potential problems are more specifically identified. Actual performance is often observed in context to identify what supports performance and what hinders performance. Performance skills, performance patterns, context or contexts, activity demands, and client factors are all considered, but only selected aspects may be specifically assessed. Targeted outcomes are identified.

■ **Intervention**

Intervention plan—A plan that will guide actions taken and that is developed in collaboration with the client. It is based on selected theories, frames of reference, and evidence. Outcomes to be targeted are confirmed.

Intervention implementation—Ongoing actions taken to influence and support improved client performance. Interventions are directed at identified outcomes. Client's response is monitored and documented.

Intervention review—A review of the implementation plan and process as well as its progress toward targeted outcomes.

■ **Outcomes (Engagement in Occupation To Support Participation)**

Outcomes—Determination of success in reaching desired targeted outcomes. Outcome assessment information is used to plan future actions with the client and to evaluate the service program (i.e., program evaluation).

Figure 2. Framework Process of Service Delivery as Applied Within the Profession's Domain.

laborative therapeutic relationship between the client and the occupational therapist and occupational therapy assistant.

To help the reader understand the process, key statements highlight important points about the process outlined below.

The process outlined is dynamic and interactive in nature. Although the parts of the Framework are described in a linear manner, in reality, the process does not occur in a sequenced, step-by-step fashion. The arrows in Figure 3 that connect the boxes indicate the interactive and nonlinear nature of the process. The process, however, does always start with the occupational profile. An understanding of the client's concerns, problems, and risks is the cornerstone of the process. The factors that influence occupational performance (performance skills, performance patterns, context or contexts, activity demands, client factors) continually interact with one another. Because of their dynamic interaction, these factors are frequently evaluated simultaneously throughout the process as their influence on performance is observed.

Context is an overarching, underlying, embedded influence on the process of service delivery. Contexts exist around and within the person. They influence both the client's performance and the process of delivering services. The external context (e.g., the physical setting, social and virtual contexts) provide resources that support or inhibit the client's performance (e.g., presence of a willing caregiver) as well as the delivery of services (e.g., limits placed on length of intervention in an inpatient hospital setting). Different settings (i.e., community, institution, home) provide different supports and resources for service

delivery. The client's internal context (personal and spiritual contexts) affects service delivery by influencing personal beliefs, perceptions, and expectations. The cultural context, which exists outside of the person but is internalized by the person, also sets expectations, beliefs, and customs that can affect how and when services may be delivered. Note that in Figure 3, context is depicted as surrounding and underlying the process.

The term *client* is used to name the entity that receives occupational therapy services. Clients may be

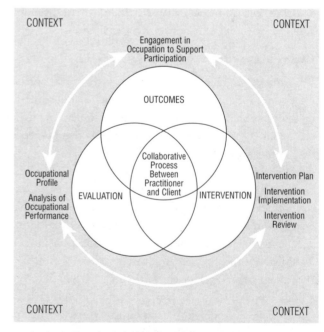

Figure 3. Framework Collaborative Process Model. Illustration of the framework emphasizing client–practitioner interactive relationship and interactive nature of the service delivery process.

categorized as (a) individuals, including individuals who may be involved in supporting or caring for the client (i.e., caregiver, teacher, parent, employer, spouse); (b) individuals within the context of a group (i.e., a family, a class); or (c) individuals within the context of a population (i.e., an organization, a community). The definition of *client* is consistent with *The Guide to Occupational Therapy Practice* (Moyers, 1999) and is indicative of the profession's growing understanding that people may be served not only as individuals, but also as members of a group or a population. The actual term used for individuals who are served will vary by practice setting. For example, in a hospital, the person might be referred to as a "patient," whereas in a school, he or she might be called a "student." Clients may be served as individuals, groups, or populations. Although the most common form of service delivery within the profession now involves a direct individual client to service provider model, more and more occupational therapists and occupational therapy assistants are beginning to serve clients at the group and population level (i.e., organization, community). When providing interventions other than in a one-to-one model, the occupational therapist and occupational therapist assistant are seen as agents who help others to support client engagement in occupations rather than as those who personally provide that support. Often, they use education and consultation as interventions. When occupational therapists and occupational therapy assistants are collaborating with clients to provide services at the group or population level, an important point to recognize is that although interventions may be directed to a group or population (i.e., organization, community), the individuals within those entities are the ones who are being evaluated and served. The wants, needs, occupational risks or problems, and performance patterns and skills of individuals within the group or population (i.e., organization, community) are evaluated as an aggregate, and information is compiled to determine group or population occupational issues and solutions.

A client-centered approach is used throughout the Framework. The Framework incorporates the value of client-centered evaluation and intervention by recognizing from the outset that all interventions must be focused on client priorities. The very nature of engagement in occupation—which is internally motivated, is individually defined, and requires active participation by the client—means that the client must be an active participant in the process. Clients identify what occupations and activities are important to them and determine the degree of engagement in each occupation. However, in some circumstances the client's ability to provide a description of the perceived or desired occupations or activity may be limited because of

either the nature of the client's problems (e.g., autism, dementia) or the stage of development (e.g., infants). When this occurs, the occupational therapist and occupational therapy assistant must then take a broader view of the client and seek input from others such as family or significant others who would have knowledge and insight into the client's desires. By involving the family or significant others, the occupational therapist and assistant can better understand the client's history, developmental stage, and current contexts. Inclusion of others in these circumstances allows the client to be represented in intervention planning and implementation.

The entire process of service delivery begins with a collaborative relationship with the client. The collaborative relationship continues throughout the process and affects all phases of the process. The central importance of this collaboration is noted in Figure 3.

The Framework is based on the belief that the occupational therapist, occupational therapy assistant, and the client bring unique resources to the Framework process. Occupational therapists and occupational therapy assistants bring knowledge about how engagement in occupation affects health and performance. They also bring knowledge about disease and disability and couple this information with their clinical reasoning and theoretical perspectives to critically observe, analyze, describe, and interpret human performance. Therapists and assistants combine their knowledge and skills to modify the factors that influence engagement in occupation to improve and support performance. Clients bring knowledge about their life experiences and their hopes and dreams for the future. Clients share their priorities, which are based on what is important to them, and collaborate with the therapist and assistant in directing the intervention process to those priorities.

"Engagement in occupation" is viewed as the overarching outcome of the occupational therapy process. The Framework emphasizes occupational therapy's unique contribution to health by identifying "engagement in occupation to support participation" as the end objective of the occupational therapy process. The profession recognizes that in some areas of practice (e.g., acute rehabilitation, hand therapy) occupational therapy intervention may focus primarily on performance skills or on client factors (i.e., body functions, body structures) that will enable engagement in occupations later in the continuum of care.

Evaluation Process

The evaluation process sets the stage for all that follows. Because occupational therapy is concerned with performance in daily life and how performance affects engagement in occupations to support participation, the evaluation process is focused on finding out what the client wants and needs to do and on identifying those factors that act as supports or barriers to performance. During the evaluation process, this information is paired with the occupational therapist's knowledge about human performance and the effect that illness, disability, and engagement in occupation have on performance. The occupational therapist considers performance skills, performance patterns, context, activity demands, and client factors and determines how each influences performance. The occupational therapist's skilled observation, use of specific assessments, and interpretation of results leads to a clear delineation of the problems and probable causes. The occupational therapy assistant may contribute to the evaluation process based on established competencies and under the supervision of an occupational therapist.

During the evaluation, a collaborative relationship with the client is established that continues throughout the entire occupational therapy process. The evaluation process is divided into two substeps, the first of which is the occupational profile—the initial step during which the client's needs, problems, and concerns about occupations and daily life activity performance are identified and priorities and values ascertained. The client's background and history in reference to engagement in occupations and in activities are also explored. The second substep of the evaluation process, analysis of occupational performance, focuses on more specifically identifying occupational performance issues and evaluating selected factors that support and hinder performance. Although each subsection is described separately and sequentially, in actuality, information pertinent to both subsections may be gathered during either one. The client's input is central in this process, and the client's priorities guide choices and decisions made during the process of evaluation.

Occupational Profile

An occupational profile is defined as information that describes the client's occupational history and experiences, patterns of daily living, interests, values, and needs. The profile is designed to gain an understanding of the client's perspective and background. Using a client-centered approach, information is gathered to understand what is currently important and meaningful to the client (what he or she wants and needs to do) and to identify past experiences and interests that may assist in the understanding of current issues and problems. During the process of collecting this information, the client's priorities and desired targeted outcomes that will lead to engagement in occupation to support participation in life are also identified. Only

clients can identify the occupations that give meaning to their lives and select the goals and priorities that are important to them. Valuing and respecting the client's input helps to foster client involvement and can more efficiently guide interventions.

Information about the occupational profile is collected at the beginning of contact with the client. However, additional information is collected over time throughout the process, refined, and reflected in changes subsequently made to targeted outcomes.

Process. The theories and frames of reference that the occupational therapist selects to guide his or her reasoning will influence the information that is collected during the occupational profile. Scientific knowledge and evidence about diagnostic conditions and occupational performance problems is used to guide information gathering.

The process of completing the occupational profile will vary depending on the setting and the client. The information gathered in the profile may be obtained both formally and informally and may be completed in one session or over a much longer period while working with the client. Obtaining information through both formal interview and casual conversation is a way of beginning to establish a therapeutic relationship with the client. Ideally, the information obtained through the occupational profile will lead to a more individualized approach in the evaluation, intervention planning, and intervention implementation stages.

Specifically, the following information is collected:
- Who is the client (individual, caregiver, group, population)?
- Why is the client seeking service, and what are the client's current concerns relative to engaging in occupations and in daily life activities?
- What areas of occupation are successful, and what areas are causing problems or risks? (see Figure 1)
- What contexts support engagement in desired occupations, and what contexts are inhibiting engagement?
- What is the client's occupational history (i.e., life experiences, values, interests, previous patterns of engagement in occupations and in daily life activities, the meanings associated with them)?
- What are the client's priorities and desired targeted outcomes (see Appendix, Table 9)?
  – Occupational performance
  – Client satisfaction
  – Role competence
  – Adaptation
  – Health and wellness
  – Prevention
  – Quality of life

After profile data are collected, the therapist reviews the information and develops a working hypothesis regarding possible reasons for identified problems and concerns and identifies the client's strengths and weaknesses. Outcome measures are preliminarily selected.

Analysis of Occupational Performance

Occupational performance is defined as the ability to carry out activities of daily life, including activities in the areas of occupation: activities of daily living (ADL) [also called basic activities of daily living (BADL) and personal activities of daily living (PADL)], instrumental activities of daily living (IADL), education, work, play, leisure, and social participation. Occupational performance results in the accomplishment of the selected occupation or activity and occurs through a dynamic transaction among the client, the context, and the activity. Improving or developing skills and patterns in occupational performance leads to engagement in one or more occupations (adapted in part from Law et al., 1996, p. 16).

When occupational performance is analyzed, the performance skills and patterns used in performance are identified, and other aspects of engaging in occupation that affect skills and patterns (e.g., client factors, activity demands, context or contexts) are evaluated. The analysis process identifies facilitators as well as barriers in various aspects of engagement in occupations and in daily life activities. Analyzing occupational performance requires an understanding of the complex and dynamic interaction among performance skills, performance patterns, context or contexts, activity demands, and client factors rather than of any one factor alone.

The information gathered during the occupational profile about the client's needs, problems, and priorities guides decisions during the analysis of occupational performance. The profile information directs the therapist's selection of the specific occupations or activities that need to be further analyzed and influences the selection of specific assessments that are used during the analysis process.

Process. Using available evidence and all aspects of clinical reasoning (scientific, narrative, pragmatic, ethical), the therapist selects one or more frames of reference to guide further collection of evaluation information. The following actions are taken:

- Synthesize information from the occupational profile to focus on specific areas of occupation and their contexts that need to be addressed.
- Observe the client's performance in desired occupations and activities, noting effectiveness of the performance skills and performance patterns. May select and use specific assessments to measure performance skills and patterns as appropriate.

- Select assessments, as needed, to identify and measure more specifically context or contexts, activity demands, and client factors that may be influencing performance skills and performance patterns.
- Interpret the assessment data to identify what supports performance and what hinders performance.
- Develop and refine hypotheses about the client's occupational performance strengths and weaknesses.
- Create goals in collaboration with the client that address the desired targeted outcomes. Confirm outcome measure to be used.
- Delineate potential intervention approach or approaches based on best practice and evidence.

Intervention Process

The intervention process is divided into three substeps: intervention plan, intervention implementation, and intervention review. During the intervention process, information from the evaluation step is integrated with theory, frames of reference, and evidence and is coupled with clinical reasoning to develop a plan and carry it out. The plan guides the actions of the occupational therapist and occupational therapy assistant and is based on the client's priorities. Interventions are carried out to address performance skills, patterns, context or contexts, activity demands, and client factors that are hindering performance. Periodic reviews throughout the process allow for revisions in the plan and actions. Again, collaboration with the client is vital in this section of the process to ensure effectiveness and success. All interventions are ultimately directed toward achieving the overarching outcome of engagement in occupation to support participation.

Intervention Plan

An intervention plan is defined as a plan that is developed based on the results of the evaluation process and describes selected occupational therapy approaches and types of interventions to reach the client's identified targeted outcomes. An intervention plan is developed collaboratively with the client (including, in some cases, family or significant others) and is based on the client's goals and priorities.

The design of the intervention plan is directed by
- the client's goals, values, and beliefs;
- the health and well-being of the client;
- the client's performance skills and performance patterns, as they are influenced by the interaction among the context or contexts, activity demands, and client factors; and
- the setting or circumstance in which the intervention is provided (e.g., caregiver expectations, organization's purpose, payer's requirements, or applicable regulations).

Interventions are designed to foster engagement in occupations and in activities to support participation in life. The selection and design of the intervention plan and goals are directed toward addressing the client's current and potential problems related to engagement in occupations or in activities.

Process. Intervention planning includes the following steps:

1. Develop the plan. The occupational therapist develops the plan. The occupational therapy assistant, based on established competencies and under the supervision of the occupational therapist, may contribute to the plan's development. The plan includes the following:
   - Objective and measurable goals with a timeframe
   - Occupational therapy intervention approach or approaches based on theory and evidence (see Appendix, Table 7).
     - Create or promote
     - Establish or restore
     - Maintain
     - Modify
     - Prevent
   - Mechanisms for service delivery
     - Who will provide intervention
     - Types of interventions
     - Frequency and duration of service
2. Consider potential discharge needs and plans.
3. Select outcome measures.
4. Make recommendation or referral to others as needed.

Intervention Implementation

Intervention is the process of putting the plan into action. Intervention implementation is defined as the skilled process of effecting change in the client's occupational performance, leading to engagement in occupations or in activities to support participation. Intervention implementation is a collaborative process between the client and the occupational therapist and assistant.

Interventions may be focused on changing the context or contexts, activity demands, client factors, performance skills, or performance patterns. Occupational therapists and occupational therapy assistants recognize that change in one factor may influence other factors. All factors that affect performance are interrelated and influence one another in a continuous dynamic process that results in performance in desired areas of occupation. Because of this dynamic interrelationship, dynamic assessment continues throughout the implementation process.

Process. Intervention implementation includes the following steps:

1. Determine and carry out the type of occupational ther-

apy intervention or interventions to be used (see Appendix, Table 8).
   - Therapeutic use of self
   - Therapeutic use of occupations or activities
     - Occupation-based activity
     - Purposeful activity
     - Preparatory methods
   - Consultation process
   - Education process
2. Monitor client's response to interventions based on ongoing assessment and reassessment.

Intervention Review

Intervention review is defined as a continuous process for reevaluating and reviewing the intervention plan, the effectiveness of its delivery, and the progress toward targeted outcomes. This process includes collaboration with the client (including, in some cases, family, significant others, and other service providers). Reevaluation and review may lead to change in the intervention plan. The intervention review process may be carried out differently in a variety of settings.

Process. The intervention review includes the following steps:

1. Reevaluate the plan and how it is carried out with the client relative to achieving targeted outcomes.
2. Modify the plan as needed.
3. Determine the need for continuation, discontinuation, or referral.

Outcomes Process

Outcomes are defined as important dimensions of health that are attributed to interventions, including ability to function, health perceptions, and satisfaction with care (adapted from Request for Planning Ideas, 2001). The important dimension of health that occupational therapists and occupational therapy assistants target as the profession's overarching outcome is "engagement in occupation to support participation." The two concepts included in this outcome are defined as follows:

- Engagement in occupation—The commitment made to performance in occupations or activities as the result of self-choice, motivation, and meaning, and includes the objective and subjective aspects of carrying out occupations and activities that are meaningful and purposeful to the person.
- Participation—"involvement in a life situation" (WHO, 2001, p. 10).

Engagement in occupation to support participation is the broad outcome of intervention that is designed to foster performance in desired and needed occupations or activities. When clients are actively involved in carrying out occupations or daily life activities that they find purposeful and meaningful in home and community settings, participation is a natural outcome. Less broad and more specific outcomes of occupational therapy intervention (see Appendix, Table 9) are multidimensional and support the end result of engagement in occupation to support participation.

In targeting engagement in occupation to support participation as the broad, overarching outcome of the occupational therapy intervention process, the profession underscores its belief that health and well-being are holistic and that they are developed and maintained through active engagement in occupation.

The focus on outcomes is interwoven throughout the process of service delivery within occupational therapy. During the evaluation phase of the process, the client's initial targeted outcomes regarding desired engagement in occupation or daily life activities are identified. As further analysis of occupational performance and development of the treatment plan take place, targeted outcomes are further refined. During intervention implementation and reevaluation, targeted outcomes may be modified based on changing needs, contexts, and performance abilities. Outcomes have numerous definitions and connotations for different clients, payers, regulators, and organizations. The specific outcomes chosen will vary by practice setting and will be influenced by the particular stakeholders in each setting.

Process. Implementation of the outcomes process includes the following steps:

1. Select types of outcomes and measures, including, but not limited to occupational performance, client satisfaction, adaptation, role competence, health and wellness, prevention, and quality of life.
   • Selection of outcome measures occurs early in the intervention process (see Evaluation Process, Occupational Profile section).
   • Outcome measures that are selected are valid, reliable, and appropriately sensitive to change in the client's occupational performance, and they match the targeted outcomes.
   • Selection of an outcome measure or instrument for a particular client should be congruent with client goals.
   • Selection of an outcome measure should entail considering its actual or purported ability to predict future outcomes.
2. Measure and use outcomes.
   • Compare progress toward goal achievement to targeted outcomes throughout the intervention process.
   • Assess outcome results and use to make decisions about future direction of intervention (i.e., continue intervention, modify intervention, discontinue intervention, provide follow-up, refer to other services).

An Overview of the Occupational Therapy Practice Process

Table 10 in the Appendix summarizes the process that occurs during occupational therapy service delivery. The arrow placed between the Occupational Profile and Analysis of Occupational Performance evaluation substeps indicates the interactions between these two. However, a similar interaction occurs among all of the steps and substeps. The process is not linear but, instead, is fluid and dynamic, allowing the occupational therapist and occupational therapy assistant to operate with an ongoing focus on outcomes while continually reflecting and changing an overall plan to accommodate new developments and insights along the way.

Acknowledgments

The Commission on Practice (COP) would like to thank and acknowledge all those who participated in the review and comment process associated with the development of the *Occupational Therapy Practice Framework: Domain and Process.* The COP has found this process invaluable and enriching. Everyone's input has been carefully reviewed and considered. Often, small comments repeated by many can lead to significant discussion and change. The COP hopes that all those who contributed to this process will continue to do so for future documents and will encourage others to participate. The profession is richer for this process.

The COP would like to thank the following individuals for their significant contributions to the direction and final content of this document: Carolyn Baum, PhD, OTR, FAOTA; Elizabeth Crepeau, PhD, OTR, FAOTA; Patricia A. Crist, PhD, FAOTA; Winifred Dunn, PhD, OTR, FAOTA; Anne G. Fisher, PhD, OTR, FAOTA; Gail S. Fidler, OTR, FAOTA; Mary Foto, OT, FAOTA; Nedra Gillette, SCD (HON), MEd, OTR, FAOTA; Jim Hinojosa, PhD, OT, FAOTA; Margo B. Holm, PhD, OTR, FAOTA; Gary Kielhofner, DRPH, OTR/L, FAOTA; Paula Kramer, PhD, OTR, FAOTA; Mary Law, PhD, OT(C); Linda T. Learnard, OTR/L; Anne Mosey, PhD, OTR, FAOTA; Penelope A. Moyers, EDd, OTR, FAOTA; David Nelson, PhD, OTR, FAOTA; Marta Pelczarski, OTR; Kathlyn L. Reed, PhD, OTR, FAOTA; Barbara Schell, PhD, OTR/L, FAOTA; Janette Schkade, PhD, OTR; Wendy Schoen; Carol Siebert, MS, OTR/L; V. Judith Thomas, MGA; Linda Kohlman Thomson, MOT, OT, OT(C), FAOTA; Amy L. Walsh, OTR/L; Wendy Wood, PhD, OTR, FAOTA; Boston University OT Students mentored by Karen Jacobs, EDd, OTR/L, CPE, FAOTA; and the University of Kansas Occupational Therapy Education Faculty.

Appendix

TABLE 1. AREAS OF OCCUPATION

Various kinds of life activities in which people engage, including ADL, IADL, education, work, play, leisure, and social participation.

■ ACTIVITIES OF DAILY LIVING (ADL)

Activities that are oriented toward taking care of one's own body (adapted from Rogers & Holm, 1994, pp. 181–202)—also called basic activities of daily living (BADL) or personal activities of daily living (PADL).

- **Bathing, showering**—Obtaining and using supplies; soaping, rinsing, and drying body parts; maintaining bathing position; and transferring to and from bathing positions.

- **Bowel and bladder management**—Includes complete intentional control of bowel movements and urinary bladder and, if necessary, use of equipment or agents for bladder control (Uniform Data System for Medical Rehabilitation [UDSMR], 1996, pp. III–20, III–24).

- **Dressing**—Selecting clothing and accessories appropriate to time of day, weather, and occasion; obtaining clothing from storage area; dressing and undressing in a sequential fashion; fastening and adjusting clothing and shoes; and applying and removing personal devices, prostheses, or orthoses.

- **Eating**—"The ability to keep and manipulate food/fluid in the mouth and swallow it (O'Sullivan, 1995, p. 191)" (AOTA, 2000, p. 629).

- **Feeding**—"The process of [setting up, arranging, and] bringing food [fluids] from the plate or cup to the mouth (O'Sullivan, 1995, p. 191)" (AOTA, 2000, p. 629).

- **Functional mobility**—Moving from one position or place to another (during performance of everyday activities), such as in-bed mobility, wheelchair mobility, transfers (wheelchair, bed, car, tub, toilet, tub/shower, chair, floor). Performing functional ambulation and transporting objects.

- **Personal device care**—Using, cleaning, and maintaining personal care items, such as hearing aids, contact lenses, glasses, orthotics, prosthetics, adaptive equipment, and contraceptive and sexual devices.

- **Personal hygiene and grooming**—Obtaining and using supplies; removing body hair (use of razors, tweezers, lotions, etc.); applying and removing cosmetics; washing, drying, combing, styling, brushing, and trimming hair; caring for nails (hands and feet); caring for skin, ears, eyes, and nose; applying deodorant; cleaning mouth; brushing and flossing teeth; or removing, cleaning, and reinserting dental orthotics and prosthetics.

- **Sexual activity**—Engagement in activities that result in sexual satisfaction.

- **Sleep/rest**—A period of inactivity in which one may or may not suspend consciousness.

- **Toilet hygiene**—Obtaining and using supplies; clothing management; maintaining toileting position; transferring to and from toileting position; cleaning body; and caring for menstrual and continence needs (including catheters, colostomies, and suppository management).

■ INSTRUMENTAL ACTIVITIES OF DAILY LIVING (IADL)

Activities that are oriented toward interacting with the environment and that are often complex—generally optional in nature (i.e., may be delegated to another) (adapted from Rogers & Holm, 1994, pp. 181–202).

- **Care of others (including selecting and supervising caregivers)**—Arranging, supervising, or providing the care for others.

- **Care of pets**—Arranging, supervising, or providing the care for pets and service animals.

- **Child rearing**—Providing the care and supervision to support the developmental needs of a child.

- **Communication device use**—Using equipment or systems such as writing equipment, telephones, typewriters, computers, communication boards, call lights, emergency systems, braille writers, telecommunication devices for the deaf, and augmentative communication systems to send and receive information.

- **Community mobility**—Moving self in the community and using public or private transportation, such as driving, or accessing buses, taxi cabs, or other public transportation systems.

- **Financial management**—Using fiscal resources, including alternate methods of financial transaction and planning and using finances with long-term and short-term goals.

- **Health management and maintenance**—Developing, managing, and maintaining routines for health and wellness promotion, such as physical fitness, nutrition, decreasing health risk behaviors, and medication routines.

- **Home establishment and management**—Obtaining and maintaining personal and household possessions and environment (e.g., home, yard, garden, appliances, vehicles), including maintaining and repairing personal possessions (clothing and household items) and knowing how to seek help or whom to contact.

- **Meal preparation and cleanup**—Planning, preparing, serving well-balanced, nutritional meals and cleaning up food and utensils after meals.

- **Safety procedures and emergency responses**—Knowing and performing preventive procedures to maintain a safe environment as well as recognizing sudden, unexpected hazardous situations and initiating emergency action to reduce the threat to health and safety.

- **Shopping**—Preparing shopping lists (grocery and other); selecting and purchasing items; selecting method of payment; and completing money transactions.

■ EDUCATION

Includes activities needed for being a student and participating in a learning environment.

- **Formal educational participation**—Including the categories of academic (e.g., math, reading, working on a degree), nonacademic (e.g., recess, lunchroom, hallway), extracurricular (e.g., sports, band, cheerleading, dances), and vocational (prevocational and vocational) participation.

- **Exploration of informal personal educational needs or interests (beyond formal education)**—Identifying topics and methods for obtaining topic-related information or skills.

- **Informal personal education participation**—Participating in classes, programs, and activities that provide instruction/training in identified areas of interest.

■ WORK

Includes activities needed for engaging in remunerative employment or volunteer activities (Mosey, 1996, p. 341).

- **Employment interests and pursuits**—Identifying and selecting work opportunities based on personal assets, limitations, likes, and dislikes relative to work (adapted from Mosey, 1996, p. 342).

- **Employment seeking and acquisition**—Identifying job opportunities, completing and submitting appropriate application materials, preparing for interviews, participating in interviews and following up afterward, discussing job benefits, and finalizing negotiations.

- **Job performance**—Including work habits, for example, attendance, punctuality, appropriate relationships with coworkers and supervisors, completion of assigned work, and compliance with the norms of the work setting (adapted from Mosey, 1996, p. 342).

- **Retirement preparation and adjustment**—Determining aptitudes, developing interests and skills, and selecting appropriate avocational pursuits.

(Continued)

TABLE 1. AREAS OF OCCUPATION

(Continued)

- **Volunteer exploration**—Determining community causes, organizations, or opportunities for unpaid "work" in relationship to personal skills, interests, location, and time available.

- **Volunteer participation**—Performing unpaid "work" activities for the benefit of identified selected causes, organizations, or facilities.

■ PLAY

"Any spontaneous or organized activity that provides enjoyment, entertainment, amusement, or diversion" (Parham & Fazio, 1997, p. 252).

- **Play exploration**—Identifying appropriate play activities, which can include exploration play, practice play, pretend play, games with rules, constructive play, and symbolic play (adapted from Bergen, 1988, pp. 64–65).

- **Play participation**—Participating in play; maintaining a balance of play with other areas of occupation; and obtaining, using, and maintaining, toys, equipment, and supplies appropriately.

■ LEISURE

"A nonobligatory activity that is intrinsically motivated and engaged in during discretionary time, that is, time not committed to obligatory occupations such as work, self-care, or sleep" (Parham & Fazio, 1997, p. 250).

- **Leisure exploration**—Identifying interests, skills, opportunities, and appropriate leisure activities.

- **Leisure participation**—Planning and participating in appropriate leisure activities; maintaining a balance of leisure activities with other areas of occupation; and obtaining, using, and maintaining equipment and supplies as appropriate.

■ SOCIAL PARTICIPATION

Activities associated with organized patterns of behavior that are characteristic and expected of an individual or an individual interacting with others within a given social system (adapted from Mosey, 1996, p. 340).

- **Community**—Activities that result in successful interaction at the community level (i.e., neighborhood, organizations, work, school).

- **Family**—"[Activities that result in] successful interaction in specific required and/or desired familial roles" (Mosey, 1996, p. 340).

- **Peer, friend**—Activities at different levels of intimacy, including engaging in desired sexual activity.

Note. Some of the terms used in this table are from, or adapted from, the rescinded *Uniform Terminology for Occupational Therapy—Third Edition* (AOTA, 1994, pp. 1047–1054).

TABLE 2. PERFORMANCE SKILLS

Features of what one does, not what one has, related to observable elements of action that have implicit functional purposes (adapted from Fisher & Kielhofner, 1995, p. 113).

■ MOTOR SKILLS—skills in moving and interacting with task, objects, and environment (A. Fisher, personal communication, July 9, 2001).

- **Posture**—Relates to the stabilizing and aligning of one's body while moving in relation to task objects with which one must deal.

Stabilizes—Maintains trunk control and balance while interacting with task objects such that there is no evidence of transient (i.e., quickly passing) propping or loss of balance that affects task performance.

Aligns—Maintains an upright sitting or standing position, without evidence of a need to persistently prop during the task performance.

Positions—Positions body, arms, or wheelchair in relation to task objects and in a manner that promotes the use of efficient arm movements during task performance.

- **Mobility**—Relates to moving the entire body or a body part in space as necessary when interacting with task objects.

Walks—Ambulates on level surfaces and changes direction while walking without shuffling the feet, lurching, instability, or using external supports or assistive devices (e.g., cane, walker, wheelchair) during the task performance.

Reaches—Extends, moves the arm (and when appropriate, the trunk) to effectively grasp or place task objects that are out of reach, including skillfully using a reacher to obtain task objects.

Bends—Actively flexes, rotates, or twists the trunk in a manner and direction appropriate to the task.

- **Coordination**—Relates to using more than one body part to interact with task objects in a manner that supports task performance.

Coordinates—Uses two or more body parts together to stabilize and manipulate task objects during bilateral motor tasks.

Manipulates—Uses dexterous grasp-and-release patterns, isolated finger movements, and coordinated in-hand manipulation patterns when interacting with task objects.

Flows—Uses smooth and fluid arm and hand movements when interacting with task objects.

- **Strength and effort**—Pertains to skills that require generation of muscle force appropriate for effective interaction with task objects.

Moves—Pushes, pulls, or drags task objects along a supporting surface.

Transports—Carries task objects from one place to another while walking, seated in a wheelchair, or using a walker.

Lifts—Raises or hoists task objects, including lifting an object from one place to another, but without ambulating or moving from one place to another.

Calibrates—Regulates or grades the force, speed, and extent of movement when interacting with task objects (e.g., not too much or too little).

Grips—Pinches or grasps task objects with no "grip slips."

- **Energy**—Refers to sustained effort over the course of task performance.

Endures—Persists and completes the task without obvious evidence of physical fatigue, pausing to rest, or stopping to "catch one's breath."

Paces—Maintains a consistent and effective rate or tempo of performance throughout the steps of the entire task.

■ PROCESS SKILLS—"Skills...used in managing and modifying actions en route to the completion of daily life tasks" (Fisher & Kielhofner, 1995, p. 120).

- **Energy**—Refers to sustained effort over the course of task performance.

Paces—Maintains a consistent and effective rate or tempo of performance throughout the steps of the entire task.

(Continued)

TABLE 2. PERFORMANCE SKILLS

(Continued)

Attends—Maintains focused attention throughout the task such that the client is not distracted away from the task by extraneous auditory or visual stimuli.

- **Knowledge**—Refers to the ability to seek and use task-related knowledge.

Chooses—Selects appropriate and necessary tools and materials for the task, including choosing the tools and materials that were specified for use prior to the initiation of the task.

Uses—Uses tools and materials according to their intended purposes and in a reasonable or hygienic fashion, given their intrinsic properties and the availability (or lack of availability) of other objects.

Handles—Supports, stabilizes, and holds tools and materials in an appropriate manner that protects them from damage, falling, or dropping.

Heeds—Uses goal-directed task actions that are focused toward the completion of the specified task (i.e., the outcome originally agreed on or specified by another) without behavior that is driven or guided by environmental cues (i.e., "environmentally cued" behavior).

Inquires—(a) Seeks needed verbal or written information by asking questions or reading directions or labels or (b) asks no unnecessary information questions (e.g., questions related to where materials are located or how a familiar task is performed).

- **Temporal organization**—Pertains to the beginning, logical ordering, continuation, and completion of the steps and action sequences of a task.

Initiates—Starts or begins the next action or step without hesitation.

Continues—Performs actions or action sequences of steps without unnecessary interruption such that once an action sequence is initiated, the individual continues on until the step is completed.

Sequences—Performs steps in an effective or logical order for efficient use of time and energy and with an absence of (a) randomness in the ordering and/or (b) inappropriate repetition ("reordering") of steps.

Terminates—Brings to completion single actions or single steps without perseveration, inappropriate persistence, or premature cessation.

- **Organizing space and objects**—Pertains to skills for organizing task spaces and task objects.

Searches/locates—Looks for and locates tools and materials in a logical manner, including looking beyond the immediate environment (e.g., looking in, behind, on top of).

Gathers—Collects together needed or misplaced tools and materials, including (a) collecting located supplies into the workspace and (b) collecting and replacing materials that have spilled, fallen, or been misplaced.

Organizes—Logically positions or spatially arranges tools and materials in an orderly fashion (a) within a single workspace and (b) among multiple appropriate workspaces to facilitate ease of task performance.

Restores—(a) Puts away tools and materials in appropriate places, (b) restores immediate workspace to original condition (e.g., wiping surfaces clean), (c) closes and seals containers and coverings when indicated, and (d) twists or folds any plastic bags to seal.

Navigates—Modifies the movement pattern of the arm, body, or wheelchair to maneuver around obstacles that are encountered in the course of moving through space such that undesirable contact with obstacles (e.g., knocking over, bumping into) is avoided (includes maneuvering objects held in the hand around obstacles).

- **Adaptation**—Relates to the ability to anticipate, correct for, and benefit by learning from the consequences of errors that arise in the course of task performance.

Notices/responds—Responds appropriately to (a) nonverbal environmental/perceptual cues (i.e., movement, sound, smell, heat, moisture, texture, shape, consistency) that provide feedback with respect to task progression and (b) the spatial arrangement of objects to one another (e.g., aligning objects during stacking). Notices and, when indicated, makes an effective and efficient response.

Accommodates—Modifies his or her actions or the location of objects within the workspace in anticipation of or in response to problems that might arise. The client anticipates or responds to problems effectively by (a) changing the method with which he or she is performing an action sequence, (b) changing the manner in which he or she interacts with or handles tools and materials already in the workspace, and (c) asking for assistance when appropriate or needed.

Adjusts—Changes working environments in anticipation of or in response to problems that might arise. The client anticipates or responds to problems effectively by making some change (a) between working environments by moving to a new workspace or bringing in or removing tools and materials from the present workspace or (b) in an environmental condition (e.g., turning on or off the tap, turning up or down the temperature).

Benefits—Anticipates and prevents undesirable circumstances or problems from recurring or persisting.

■ **COMMUNICATION/INTERACTION SKILLS**—Refer to conveying intentions and needs and coordinating social behavior to act together with people (Forsyth & Kielhofner, 1999; Forsyth, Salamy, Simon, & Kielhofner, 1997; Kielhofner, 2002).

- **Physicality**—Pertains to using the physical body when communicating within an occupation.

Contacts—Makes physical contact with others.

Gazes—Uses eyes to communicate and interact with others.

Gestures—Uses movements of the body to indicate, demonstrate, or add emphasis.

Maneuvers—Moves one's body in relation to others.

Orients—Directs one's body in relation to others and/or occupational forms.

Postures—Assumes physical positions.

- **Information exchange**—Refers to giving and receiving information within an occupation.

Articulates—Produces clear, understandable speech.

Asserts—Directly expresses desires, refusals, and requests.

Asks—Requests factual or personal information.

Engages—Initiates interactions.

Expresses—Displays affect/attitude.

Modulates—Uses volume and inflection in speech.

Shares—Gives out factual or personal information.

Speaks—Makes oneself understood through use of words, phrases, and sentences.

Sustains—Keeps up speech for appropriate duration.

- **Relations**—Relates to maintaining appropriate relationships within an occupation.

Collaborates—Coordinates action with others toward a common end goal.

Conforms—Follows implicit and explicit social norms.

Focuses—Directs conversation and behavior to ongoing social action.

Relates—Assumes a manner of acting that tries to establish a rapport with others.

Respects—Accommodates to other people's reactions and requests.

Note. The Motor and Process Skills sections of this table were compiled from the following sources: Fisher (2001), Fisher and Kielhofner (1995)—updated by Fisher (2001). The Communication/Interaction Skills section of this table was compiled from the following sources: Forsyth and Kielhofner (1999), Forsyth, Salamy, Simon, and Kielhofner (1997), and Kielhofner (2002).

TABLE 3. PERFORMANCE PATTERNS

Patterns of behavior related to daily life activities that are habitual or routine.

■ **HABITS**—"Automatic behavior that is integrated into more complex patterns that enable people to function on a day-to-day basis" (Neistadt & Crepeau, 1998, p. 869). Habits can either support or interfere with performance in areas of occupation.

Type of Habit	Examples
• **Useful habits**	
Habits that support performance in daily life and contribute to life satisfaction.	– Always put car keys in the same place so they can be found easily.
Habits that support ability to follow rhythms of daily life.	– Brush teeth every morning to maintain good oral hygiene.
• **Impoverished habits**	
Habits that are not established.	– Inconsistently remembering to look both ways before crossing the street.
Habits that need practice to improve.	– Inability to complete all steps of a self-care routine.
• **Dominating habits**	
Habits that are so demanding they interfere with daily life.	– Repetitive self-stimulation such as type occurring in autism.
	– Use of chemical substances, resulting in addiction.
Habits that satisfy a compulsive need for order.	– Neatly arranging forks on top of each other in silverware drawer.

■ **ROUTINES**—"Occupations with established sequences" (Christiansen & Baum, 1997, p. 6).

■ **ROLES**—"A set of behaviors that have some socially agreed upon function and for which there is an accepted code of norms" (Christiansen & Baum, 1997, p. 603).

Note. Information for Habits section of this table adapted from Dunn (2000, Fall).

TABLE 4. CONTEXT OR CONTEXTS

Context (including cultural, physical, social, personal, spiritual, temporal, and virtual) refers to a variety of interrelated conditions within and surrounding the client that influence performance.

Context	Definition	Example
Cultural	Customs, beliefs, activity patterns, behavior standards, and expectations accepted by the society of which the individual is a member. Includes political aspects, such as laws that affect access to resources and affirm personal rights. Also includes opportunities for education, employment, and economic support.	• Ethnicity, family, attitude, beliefs, values
Physical	Nonhuman aspects of contexts. Includes the accessibility to and performance within environments having natural terrain, plants, animals, buildings, furniture, objects, tools, or devices.	• Objects, built environment, natural environment, geographic terrain, sensory qualities of environment
Social	Availability and expectations of significant individuals, such as spouse, friends, and caregivers. Also includes larger social groups that are influential in establishing norms, role expectations, and social routines.	• Relationships with individuals, groups, or organizations; relationships with systems (political, economic, institutional)
Personal	"[F]eatures of the individual that are not part of a health condition or health status" (WHO, 2001, p. 17). Personal context includes age, gender, socioeconomic status, and educational status.	• Twenty-five-year-old unemployed man with a high school diploma
Spiritual	The fundamental orientation of a person's life; that which inspires and motivates that individual.	• Essence of the person, greater or higher purpose, meaning, substance
Temporal	"Location of occupational performance in time" (Neistadt & Crepeau, 1998, p. 292).	• Stages of life, time of day, time of year, duration
Virtual	Environment in which communication occurs by means of airways or computers and an absence of physical contact.	• Realistic simulation of an environment, chat rooms, radio transmissions

Note. Some of the definitions for areas of context or contexts are from the rescinded *Uniform Terminology for Occupational Therapy—Third Edition* (AOTA, 1994).

TABLE 5. ACTIVITY DEMANDS

The aspects of an activity, which include the objects, space, social demands, sequencing or timing, required actions, and required underlying body functions and body structure needed to carry out the activity.

Activity Demand Aspects	Definition	Examples
Objects and their properties	The tools, materials, and equipment used in the process of carrying out the activity	• Tools (scissors, dishes, shoes, volleyball) • Materials (paints, milk, lipstick) • Equipment (workbench, stove, basketball hoop) • Inherent properties (heavy, rough, sharp, colorful, loud, bitter tasting)
Space demands (relates to physical context)	The physical environmental requirements of the activity (e.g., size, arrangement, surface, lighting, temperature, noise, humidity, ventilation)	• Large open space outdoors required for a baseball game
Social demands (relates to social and cultural contexts)	The social structure and demands that may be required by the activity	• Rules of game • Expectations of other participants in activity (e.g., sharing of supplies)
Sequence and timing	The process used to carry out the activity (specific steps, sequence, timing requirements)	• Steps—to make tea: gather cup and tea bag, heat water, pour water into cup, etc. • Sequence—heat water before placing tea bag in water • Timing—leave tea bag to steep for 2 minutes
Required actions	The usual skills that would be required by any performer to carry out the activity. Motor, process, and communication interaction skills should each be considered. The performance skills demanded by an activity will be correlated with the demands of the other activity aspects (i.e., objects, space)	• Gripping handlebar • Choosing a dress from closet • Answering a question
Required body functions	"The physiological functions of body systems (including psychological functions)" (WHO, 2001, p. 10) that are required to support the actions used to perform the activity.	• Mobility of joints • Level of consciousness
Required body structures	"Anatomical parts of the body such as organs, limbs, and their components [that support body function]" (WHO, 2001, p. 10) that are required to perform the activity.	• Number of hands • Number of eyes

TABLE 6. CLIENT FACTORS

Those factors that reside within the client and that may affect performance in areas of occupation. Client factors include body functions and body structures. Knowledge about body functions and structures is considered when determining which functions and structures are needed to carry out an occupation/activity and how the body functions and structures may be changed as a result of engaging in an occupation/activity. Body functions are "the physiological functions of body systems (including psychological functions)" (WHO, 2001, p. 10). Body structures are "anatomical parts of the body such as organs, limbs and their components [that support body function]" (WHO, 2001, p. 10).

Client Factor	Selected Classifications From ICF and Occupational Therapy Examples
■ **BODY FUNCTION CATEGORIES**[a]	
Mental functions (affective, cognitive, perceptual)	
• Global mental functions	*Consciousness functions*—level of arousal, level of consciousness.
	Orientation functions—to person, place, time, self, and others.
	Sleep—amount and quality of sleep. *Note:* Sleep and sleep patterns are assessed in relation to how they affect ability to effectively engage in occupations and in daily life activities.
	Temperament and personality functions—conscientiousness, emotional stability, openness to experience. *Note:* These functions are assessed relative to their influence on the ability to engage in occupations and in daily life activities.
	Energy and drive functions—motivation, impulse control, interests, values.
• Specific mental functions	*Attention functions*—sustained attention, divided attention.
	Memory functions—retrospective memory, prospective memory.
	Perceptual functions—visuospatial perception, interpretation of sensory stimuli (tactile, visual, auditory, olfactory, gustatory).
	Thought functions—recognition, categorization, generalization, awareness of reality, logical/coherent thought, appropriate thought content.

(Continued)

TABLE 6. CLIENT FACTORS

(Continued)

Client Factor	Selected Classifications From ICF and Occupational Therapy Examples
	Higher-level cognitive functions—judgment, concept formation, time management, problem solving, decision-making.
	Mental functions of language—able to receive language and express self through spoken and written or sign language. *Note:* This function is assessed relative to its influence on the ability to engage in occupations and in daily life activities.
	Calculation functions—able to add or subtract. *Note:* These functions are assessed relative to their influence on the ability to engage in occupations and in daily life activities (e.g., making change when shopping).
	Mental functions of sequencing complex movement—motor planning.
	Psychomotor functions—appropriate range and regulation of motor response to psychological events.
	Emotional functions—appropriate range and regulation of emotions, self-control.
	Experience of self and time functions—body image, self-concept, self-esteem.
Sensory functions and pain	
• Seeing and related functions	*Seeing functions*—visual acuity, visual field functions.
• Hearing and vestibular functions	*Hearing function*—response to sound. *Note:* This function is assessed in terms of its presence or absence and its affect on engaging in occupations and in daily life activities.
	Vestibular function—balance.
• Additional sensory functions	*Taste function*—ability to discriminate tastes.
	Smell function—ability to discriminate smell.
	Proprioceptive function—kinesthesia, joint position sense.
	Touch functions—sensitivity to touch, ability to discriminate.
	Sensory functions related to temperature and other stimuli—sensitivity to temperature, sensitivity to pressure, ability to discriminate temperature and pressure.
• Pain	*Sensations of pain*—dull pain, stabbing pain.
Neuromusculoskeletal and movement-related functions	
• Functions of joints and bones	*Mobility of joint functions*—passive range of motion.
	Stability of joint functions—postural alignment. *Note:* This refers to physiological stability of the joint related to its structural integrity as compared to the motor skill of aligning the body while moving in relation to task objects.
	Mobility of bone functions—frozen scapula, movement of carpal bones.
• Muscle functions	*Muscle power functions*—strength.
	Muscle tone functions—degree of muscle tone (e.g., flaccidity, spasticity).
	Muscle endurance functions—endurance.
• Movement functions	*Motor reflex functions*—stretch reflex, asymmetrical tonic neck reflex.
	Involuntary movement reaction functions—righting reactions, supporting reactions.
	Control of voluntary movement functions—eye–hand coordination, bilateral integration, eye–foot coordination.
	Involuntary movement functions—tremors, tics, motor perseveration.
	Gait pattern functions—walking patterns and impairments, such as asymmetric gait, stiff gait. (*Note:* Gait patterns are assessed in relation to how they affect ability to engage in occupations and in daily life activities.)
Cardiovascular, hematological, immunological, and respiratory system function	
• Cardiovascular system function	*Blood pressure functions*—hypertension, hypotension, postural hypotension.
• Hematological and immunological system function	Occupational therapists and occupational therapy assistants have knowledge of these body functions and understand broadly the interaction that occurs between these functions and engagement in occupation to support participation. Some therapists may specialize in evaluating and intervening with a specific function as it is related to supporting performance and engagement in occupations and activities targeted for intervention.

(Continued)

TABLE 6. CLIENT FACTORS

(Continued)

Client Factor	Selected Classifications From ICF and Occupational Therapy Examples
• Respiratory system function	*Respiration functions*—rate, rhythm, and depth.
• Additional functions and sensations of the cardiovascular and respiratory systems	*Exercise tolerance functions*—physical endurance, aerobic capacity, stamina, and fatigability.

Voice and speech functions
Digestive, metabolic, and endocrine system function
  • Digestive system function
  • Metabolic system and endocrine system function
 	
Genitourinary and reproductive functions
  • Urinary functions
  • Genital and reproductive functions
	Occupational therapists and occupational therapy assistants have knowledge of these body functions and understand broadly the interaction that occurs between these functions and engagement in occupation to support participation. Some therapists may specialize in evaluating and intervening with a specific function as it is related to supporting performance and engagement in occupations and activities targeted for intervention.

Skin and related structure functions
  • Skin functions
 	
  • Hair and nail functions
	Protective functions of the skin—presence or absence of wounds, cuts, or abrasions.
	Repair function of the skin—wound healing.
	Occupational therapists and occupational therapy assistants have knowledge of these body functions and understand broadly the interaction that occurs between these functions and engagement in occupation to support participation. Some therapists may specialize in evaluating and intervening with a specific function as it is related to supporting performance and engagement in occupations and activities targeted for intervention.

Client Factor	Classifications (Classification are not delineated in the Body Structure section of this table)
■ **BODY STRUCTURE CATEGORIES**[b]	
Structure of the nervous system **The eye, ear, and related structures** **Structures involved in voice and speech** **Structures of the cardiovascular, immunological, and respiratory systems** **Structures related to the digestive** **Structure related to the genitourinary and reproductive systems** **Structures related to movement** **Skin and related structures**	Occupational therapists and occupational therapy assistants have knowledge of these body functions and understand broadly the interaction that occurs between these structures and engagement in occupation to support participation. Some therapists may specialize in evaluating and intervening with a specific structures as it is related to supporting performance and engagement in occupations and activities targeted for intervention.

Note. The reader is strongly encouraged to use *International Classification of Functioning, Disability and Health* (ICF) in collaboration with this table to provide for in-depth information with respect to classification in terms (inclusion and exclusion).

[a]Categories and classifications are adapted from the ICF (WHO, 2001). [b]Categories are from the ICF (WHO, 2001).

TABLE 7. OCCUPATIONAL THERAPY INTERVENTION APPROACHES

Specific strategies selected to direct the process of intervention that are based on the client's desired outcome, evaluation data, and evidence.

Approach	Focus of Intervention	Examples
Create, promote (health promotion)[a]—an intervention approach that does not assume a disability is present or that any factors would interfere with performance. This approach is designed to provide enriched contextual and activity experiences that will enhance performance for all persons in the natural contexts of life (adapted from Dunn, McClain, Brown, & Youngstrom, 1998, p. 534).	**Performance skills**	• Create a parenting class for first-time parents to teach child development information (performance skill).
	Performance patterns	• Promote handling stress by creating time-use routines with healthy clients (performance pattern).
	Context or contexts	• Create a variety of equipment available at public playgrounds to promote a diversity of sensory play experiences (context).
	Activity demands	• Promote the establishment of sufficient space to allow senior residents to participate in congregate cooking (activity demand).
	Client factors (body functions, body structures)	• Promote increased endurance in school children by having them ride bicycles to school (client factor: body function).
Establish, restore (remediation, restoration)[a]—an intervention approach designed to change client variables to establish a skill or ability that has not yet developed or to restore a skill or ability that has been impaired (adapted from Dunn et al., 1998, p. 533).	**Performance skills**	• Improve coping needed for changing workplace demands by improving assertiveness skills (performance skill).
	Performance patterns	• Establish morning routines needed to arrive at school or work on time (performance pattern).
	Client factors (body functions, body structures)	• Restore mobility needed for play activities (client factor: body function).
Maintain—an intervention approach designed to provide the supports that will allow clients to preserve their performance capabilities that they have regained, that continue to meet their occupational needs, or both. The assumption is that without continued maintenance intervention, performance would decrease, occupational needs would not be met, or both, thereby affecting health and quality of life.	**Performance skills**	• Maintain the ability to organize tools by providing a tool outline painted on a pegboard (performance skill).
	Performance patterns	• Maintain appropriate medication schedule by providing a timer (performance pattern).
	Context or contexts	• Maintain safe and independent access for persons with low vision by providing increased hallway lighting (context).
	Activity demands	• Maintain independent gardening for persons with arthritic hands by providing tools with modified grips (activity demand).
	Client factors (body functions, body structures)	• Maintain proper digestive system functions by developing a dining program (client factor: body function). • Maintain upper-extremity muscles necessary for independent wheelchair mobility by developing an after-school–based exercise program (client factor: body structure).
Modify (compensation, adaptation)[a]—an intervention approach directed at "finding ways to revise the current context or activity demands to support performance in the natural setting…[includes] compensatory techniques, including enhancing some features to provide cues, or reducing other features to reduce distractibility" (Dunn et al., 1998, p. 533).	**Context or contexts**	• Modify holiday celebration activities to exclude alcohol to support sobriety (context).
	Activity demands	• Modify office equipment (e.g. chair, computer station) to support individual employee body function and performance skill abilities (activity demand).
	Performance patterns	• Modify daily routines to provide consistency and predictability to support individual's cognitive ability (performance pattern).
Prevent (disability prevention)[a]—an intervention approach designed to address clients with or without a disability who are at risk for occupational performance problems. This approach is designed to prevent the occurrence or evolution of barriers to performance in context. Interventions may be directed at client, context, or activity variables (adapted from Dunn et al., 1998, p. 534).	**Performance skills**	• Prevent poor posture when sitting for prolonged periods by providing a chair with proper back support (performance skill).
	Performance patterns	• Prevent the use of chemical substances by introducing self-initiated strategies to assist in remaining drug free (performance pattern).
	Context or contexts	• Prevent social isolation by suggesting participation in after-work group activities (context).
	Activity demands	• Prevent back injury by providing instruction in proper lifting techniques (activity demand).
	Client factors (body functions, body structures)	• Prevent increased blood pressure during homemaking activities by learning to monitor blood pressure in a cardiac exercise program (client factor: body function). • Prevent repetitive stress injury by suggesting that a wrist support splint be worn when typing (client factor: body structure).

[a]Parallel language used in Moyers (1999, p. 274).

TABLE 8. TYPES OF OCCUPATIONAL THERAPY INTERVENTIONS

THERAPEUTIC USE OF SELF—A practitioner's planned use of his or her personality, insights, perceptions, and judgments as part of the therapeutic process (adapted from Punwar & Peloquin, 2000, p. 285).

THERAPEUTIC USE OF OCCUPATIONS AND ACTIVITIES[a]—Occupations and activities selected for specific clients that meet therapeutic goals. To use occupations/activities therapeutically, context or contexts, activity demands, and client factors all should be considered in relation to the client's therapeutic goals.

Occupation-based activity	*Purpose:* Allows clients to engage in actual occupations that are part of their own context and that match their goals.
	Examples:
	• Play on playground equipment during recess.
	• Purchase own groceries and prepare a meal.
	• Adapt the assembly line to achieve greater safety.
	• Put on clothes without assistance.
Purposeful activity	*Purpose:* Allows the client to engage in goal-directed behaviors or activities within a therapeutically designed context that lead to an occupation or occupations.
	Examples:
	• Practice vegetable slicing.
	• Practice drawing a straight line.
	• Practice safe ways to get in and out of a bathtub equipped with grab bars.
	• Role play to learn ways to manage anger.
Preparatory methods	*Purpose:* Prepares the client for occupational performance. Used in preparation for purposeful and occupation-based activities.
	Examples:
	• Sensory input to promote optimum response
	• Physical agent modalities
	• Orthotics/splinting (design, fabrication, application)
	• Exercise

CONSULTATION PROCESS—A type of intervention in which practitioners use their knowledge and expertise to collaborate with the client. The collaborative process involves identifying the problem, creating possible solutions, trying solutions, and altering them as necessary for greater effectiveness. When providing consultation, the practitioner is not directly responsible for the outcome of the intervention (Dunn, 2000, p. 113).

EDUCATION PROCESS—An intervention process that involves the imparting of knowledge and information about occupation and activity and that does not result in the actual performance of the occupation/activity.

[a]Information adapted from Pedretti and Early (2001).

TABLE 9. TYPES OF OUTCOMES

The examples listed specify how the broad outcome of engagement in occupation may be operationalized. The examples are not intended to be all-inclusive.

Outcome	Description
Occupational performance	The ability to carry out activities of daily life (areas of occupation). Occupational performance can be addressed in two different ways:
	• Improvement—used when a performance deficit is present, often as a result of an injury or disease process. This approach results in increased independence and function in ADL, IADL, education, work, play, leisure, or social participation.
	• Enhancement—used when a performance deficit is not currently present. This approach results in the development of performance skills and performance patterns that augment performance or prevent potential problems from developing in daily life occupations.
Client satisfaction	The client's affective response to his or her perceptions of the process and benefits of receiving occupational therapy services (adapted from Maciejewski, Kawiecki, & Rockwood, 1997).
Role competence	The ability to effectively meet the demand of roles in which the client engages.
Adaptation	"A change a person makes in his or her response approach when that person encounters an occupational challenge. This change is implemented when the individual's customary response approaches are found inadequate for producing some degree of mastery over the challenge" (Schultz & Schkade, 1997, p. 474).
Health and wellness	*Health*—"A complete state of physical, mental, and social well-being and not just the absence of disease or infirmity"(WHO, 1947, p. 29).
	Wellness—The condition of being in good health, including the appreciation and the enjoyment of health. Wellness is more than a lack of disease symptoms; it is a state of mental and physical balance and fitness (adapted from *Taber's Cyclopedic Medical Dictionary*, 1997, p. 2110).
Prevention	Promoting a healthy lifestyle at the individual, group, organizational, community (societal), and governmental or policy level (adapted from Brownson & Scaffa, 2001).
Quality of life	A person's dynamic appraisal of his or her life satisfactions (perceptions of progress toward one's goals), self-concept (the composite of beliefs and feelings about oneself), health and functioning (including health status, self-care capabilities, role competence), and socioeconomic factors (e.g., vocation, education, income) (adapted from Radomski, 1995; Zhan, 1992).

Note. ADL = activities of daily living; IADL = instrumental activities of daily living.

TABLE 10. OCCUPATIONAL THERAPY PRACTICE FRAMEWORK PROCESS SUMMARY

Evaluation		Intervention			Outcomes
Occupational Profile ◄──►	*Analysis of Occupational Performance*	*Intervention Plan*	*Intervention Implementation*	*Intervention Review*	*Engagement in Occupation to Support Participation*

• Who is the client?
 	
• Why is the client seeking services?
 	
• What occupations and activities are successful or are causing problems?
 	
• What contexts support or inhibit desired outcomes?
 	
• What is the client's occupational history?
 	
• What are the client's priorities and targeted outcomes?
	• Synthesize information from the occupational profile.
	
	• Observe client's performance in desired occupation/activity.
	
	• Note the effectiveness of performance skills and patterns and select assessments to identify factors (context or contexts, activity demands, client factors) that may be influencing performance skills and patterns.
	
	• Interpret assessment data to identify facilitators and barriers to performance.
	
	• Develop and refine hypotheses about client's occupational performance strengths and weaknesses.
	
	• Collaborate with client to create goals that address targeted outcomes.
	
	• Delineate areas for intervention based on best practice and evidence.
		• Develop plan that includes
		  – objective and measurable goals with timeframe,
		  – occupational therapy intervention approach based on theory and evidence, and
		  – mechanisms for service delivery.
		
		• Consider discharge needs and plan.
		
		• Select outcome measures.
		
		• Make recommendation or referral to others as needed.
			• Determine types of occupational therapy interventions to be used and carry them out.
			
			• Monitor client's response according to ongoing assessment and reassessment.
				• Reevaluate plan relative to achieving targeted outcomes.
				
				• Modify plan as needed.
				
				• Determine need for continuation, discontinuation, or referral.
					• Focus on outcomes as they relate to engagement in occupation to support participation.
					
					• Select outcome measures.
					
					• Measure and use outcomes.

◄─────────── Continue to renegotiate intervention plans and targeted outcomes. ───────────►

◄─────────── Ongoing interaction among evaluation, intervention, and outcomes occurs throughout the process. ───────────►

Glossary

A

Activities of daily living or ADL (an area of occupation)

Activities that are oriented toward taking care of one's own body (adapted from Rogers & Holm, 1994, pp. 181–202). (See Appendix, Table 1, for definitions of terms.) **ADL** is also referred to as basic activities of daily living (BADL) and personal activities of daily living (PADL).

• Bathing, showering

• Bowel and bladder management

• Dressing

• Eating

• Feeding

• Functional mobility

• Personal device care

• Personal hygiene and grooming

• Sexual activity

• Sleep/rest

• Toilet hygiene

Activity (activities)

A term that describes a class of human actions that are goal directed.

Activity demands

The aspects of an activity, which include the objects, space, social demands, sequencing or timing, required actions, and required underlying body functions and body structures needed to carry out the activity. (See Appendix, Table 5, for definitions of these aspects.)

Adaptation (as used as an outcome; see Appendix, Table 9)

"A change a person makes in his or her response approach when that person encounters an occupational challenge. This change is implemented when the individual's customary response approaches are found inadequate for producing some degree of mastery over the challenge" (Schultz & Schkade, 1997, p. 474).

Adaptation (as used as a performance skill; see Appendix, Table 2)

Relates to the ability to anticipate, correct for, and benefit by learning from the consequences of errors that arise in the course of task performance (Fisher, 2001; Fisher & Kielhofner, 1995—updated by Fisher [2001].

Areas of occupations

Various kinds of life activities in which people engage, including the following categories: ADL, IADL, education, work, play, leisure, and social participation. (See Appendix, Table 1, for definitions of terms.)

Assessment

"Shall be used to refer to specific tools or instruments that are used during the evaluation process" (AOTA, 1995, pp. 1072–1073).

B

Body functions (a client factor, including physical, cognitive, psychosocial aspects)

"The physiological functions of body systems (including psychological functions)" (WHO, 2001, p. 10). (See Appendix, Table 6, for categories.)

Body structures (a client factor)

"Anatomical parts of the body such as organs, limbs and their components [that support body function]" (WHO, 2001, p. 10). (See Appendix, Table 6, for categories.)

C

Client

(a) Individuals (including others involved in the individual's life who may also help or be served indirectly such as caregiver, teacher, parent, employer, spouse), (b) groups, or (c) populations (i.e., organizations, communities).

Client-centered approach

An orientation that honors the desires and priorities of clients in designing and implementing interventions (adapted from Dunn, 2000, p. 4).

Client factors

Those factors that reside within the client and that may affect performance in areas of occupation. Client factors include body functions and body structures. (See Appendix, Table 6, for categories.)

Client satisfaction

The client's affective response to his or her perceptions of the process and benefits of receiving occupational therapy services (adapted from Maciejewski, Kawiecki, & Rockwood, 1997, pp. 67–89).

Communication/interaction skills (a performance skill)

Refer to conveying intentions and needs as well as coordinating social behavior to act together with people (Forsyth & Kielhofner, 1999; Forsyth, Salamy, Simon, & Kielhofner, 1997; Kielhofner, 2002). (See Appendix, Table 2, for skills.)

Context or contexts

Refers to a variety of interrelated conditions within and surrounding the client that influence performance. Contexts include cultural, physical, social, personal, spiritual, temporal, and virtual. (See Appendix, Table 4, for definitions of terms.)

Cultural (a context)

"Customs, beliefs, activity patterns, behavior standards, and expectations accepted by the society of which the individual is a member. Includes political aspects, such as laws that affect access to resources and affirm personal rights. Also includes opportunities for education, employment, and economic support" (AOTA, 1994, p. 1054).

D

Dynamic assessment

Describes a process used during intervention implementation for testing the hypotheses generated through the evaluation process. Allows for evaluation of change and intervention effectiveness during intervention. Assesses the interactions among the person, environment, and activity to understand how the client learns and approaches activities. May lead to adjustments in intervention plan (adapted from Primeau & Ferguson, 1999, p. 503).

E

Education (an area of occupation)

Includes activities needed for being a student and participating in a learning environment. (See Appendix, Table 1, for definitions of terms.)

- Formal educational participation
- Informal personal educational needs or interests exploration (beyond formal education)
- Informal personal education participation

Engagement in occupation

This term recognizes the commitment made to performance in occupations or activities as the result of self-choice, motivation, and meaning and alludes to the objective and subjective aspects of being involved in and carrying out occupations and activities that are meaningful and purposeful to the person.

Evaluation

"Shall be used to refer to the process of obtaining and interpreting data necessary for intervention. This includes planning for and documenting the evaluation process and results" (AOTA, 1995, p. 1072).

G

Goals

"The result or achievement toward which effort is directed; aim; end" (*Random House Webster's College Dictionary,* 1995).

H

Habits (a performance pattern)

"Automatic behavior that is integrated into more complex patterns that enable people to function on a day-to-day basis…" (Neistadt & Crepeau, 1998, p. 869). Habits can either support or interfere with performance in areas of occupation. (See Appendix, Table 3, for descriptions of types of habits.)

Health

"A complete state of physical, mental, and social well-being and not just the absence of disease or infirmity" (WHO, 1947, p. 29).

Health status

A condition in which one successfully and satisfactorily performs occupations (adapted from McColl, Law, & Stewart, 1993, p. 5).

I

Identity

"A composite definition of the self and includes an interpersonal aspect (e.g., our roles and relationships, such as mother, wives, occupational therapists), an aspect of possibility or potential (who we *might* become), and a values aspect (that suggests importance and provides a stable basis for choices and decisions).… Identity can be viewed as the superordinate view of ourselves that includes both self-esteem and self-concept, but also importantly reflects and is influenced by the larger social world in which we find ourselves" (Christiansen, 1999, pp. 548–549).

Independence

"Having adequate resources to accomplish everyday tasks" (Christiansen & Baum, 1997, p. 597). "The profession views independence as the ability to self-determine activity performance, regardless of who actually performs the activity" (AOTA, 1994, p. 1051).

Instrumental activities of daily living or IADL (an area of occupation)

Activities that are oriented toward interacting with the environment and that are often complex. IADL are generally optional in nature, that is, may be delegated to another (adapted from Rogers & Holm, 1994, pp. 181–202). (See Appendix, Table 1, for definitions of terms.)

- Care of others (including selecting and supervising caregivers)
- Care of pets
- Child rearing
- Communication device use
- Community mobility
- Financial management
- Health management and maintenance
- Home establishment and management
- Meal preparation and cleanup
- Safety procedures and emergency responses
- Shopping

Interests

"Disposition to find pleasure and satisfaction in occupations and the self-knowledge of our enjoyment of occupations" (Kielhofner, Borell, Burke, Helfrick, & Nygard, 1995, p. 47).

Intervention approaches

Specific strategies selected to direct the process of interventions that are based on the client's desired outcome, evaluation date, and evidence. (See Appendix, Table 7, for definitions of various occupational therapy intervention approaches.) The terms in parentheses indicate parallel language used in Moyers (1999, p. 274).

- Create/promote (health promotion)
- Establish/restore (remediation/restoration)
- Maintain
- Modify (compensation/adaptation)
- Prevent (disability prevention)

Intervention implementation

The skilled process of effecting change in the client's occupational performance leading to engagement in occupations or activities to support participation.

Intervention plan

An outline of selected approaches and types of interventions, which is based on the results of the evaluation process, developed to reach the client's identified targeted outcomes.

Intervention review

A continuous process for reevaluating and reviewing the intervention plan, the effectiveness of implementation, and the progress toward targeted outcomes.

Interventions

(See Appendix, Table 8, for definitions of the types of occupational therapy interventions.)

- Therapeutic use of self
- Therapeutic use of occupations/activities
- Consultation process
- Education process

L

Leisure (an area of occupation)

"A nonobligatory activity that is intrinsically motivated and engaged in during discretionary time, that is, time not committed to obligatory occupations such as work, self-care, or sleep" (Parham & Fazio, 1997, p. 250). (See Appendix, Table 1, for definitions of terms.)

- Leisure exploration
- Leisure participation

M

Motor skills (a performance skill)

Skills in moving and interacting with task, objects, and environment (A. Fisher, personal communication, July 9, 2001).

O

Occupation

"Activities…of everyday life, named, organized, and given value and meaning by individuals and a culture. Occupation is everything people do to occupy themselves, including looking after themselves…enjoying life…and contributing to the social and economic fabric of their communities.…" (Law, Polatajko, Baptiste, & Townsend, 1997, p. 34).

Occupational performance

The ability to carry out activities of daily life. Includes activities in the areas of occupation: ADL (also called BADL and PADL), IADL, education, work, play, leisure, and social participation. Occupational performance is the accomplishment of the selected activity or occupation resulting from the dynamic transaction among the client, the context, and the activity. Improving or enabling skills and patterns in occupational performance leads to engagement in occupations or activities. (Adapted in part from Law et al., 1996, p. 16.)

Occupational profile

A profile that describes the client's occupational history, patterns of daily living, interests, values, and needs.

Outcomes

Important dimensions of health attributed to interventions, including ability to function, health perceptions, and satisfaction with care (adapted from Request for Planning Ideas, 2001).

P

Participation

"Involvement in a life situation" (WHO, 2001, p. 10).

Performance patterns

Patterns of behavior related to daily life activities that are habitual or routine. Performance patterns include habits and routines. (See Appendix, Table 3, for descriptions of terms.)

Performance skills

Features of what one does, not of what one has, related to observable elements of action that have implicit functional purposes (adapted from Fisher & Kielhofner, 1995, p. 113). Performance skills include motor skills, process skills, and communication/interaction skills. (See Appendix, Table 2, for definitions of skills.)

Personal (a context)

"Features of the individual that are not part of a health condition or health status" (WHO, 2001, p. 17). Personal context includes age, gender, socioeconomic status, and educational status.

Physical (a context)

"Nonhuman aspects of contexts. Includes the accessibility to and performance within environments having natural terrain, plants, animals, buildings, furniture, objects, tools, or devices" (AOTA, 1994, p. 1054).

Play (an area of occupation)

"Any spontaneous or organized activity that provides enjoyment, entertainment, amusement, or diversion" (Parham & Fazio, 1997, p. 252). (See Appendix, Table 1, for definitions of terms.)

• Play exploration

• Play participation

Prevention

Promoting a healthy lifestyle at the individual, group, organizational, community (societal), governmental/policy level (adapted from Brownson & Scaffa, 2001).

Process skills (a performance skill)

"Skills … used in managing and modifying actions en route to the completion of daily life tasks" (Fisher & Kielhofner, 1995, p. 120).

Purposeful activity

"An activity used in treatment that is goal directed and that the …[client] sees as meaningful or purposeful" (Low, 2002).

Q

Quality of life

A person's dynamic appraisal of his or her life satisfactions (perceptions of progress toward one's goals), self-concept (the composite of beliefs and feelings about oneself), health and functioning (including health status, self-care capabilities, and role competence), and socioeconomic factors (e.g., vocation, education, income) (adapted from Radomski, 1995; Zhan, 1992).

R

Reevaluation

A reassessment of the client's performance and goals to determine the type and amount of change.

Role competence

The ability to effectively meet the demand of roles in which the client engages.

Role(s)

"A set of behaviors that have some socially agreed upon function and for which there is an accepted code of norms" (Christiansen & Baum, 1997, p. 603).

Routines (a performance pattern)

"Occupations with established sequences" (Christiansen & Baum, 1997, p. 16).

S

Self-efficacy

"People's beliefs in their capabilities to organize and execute the courses of action required to deal with prospective situations" (Bandura, 1995, as cited in Rowe & Kahn, 1997, p. 437).

Social (a context)

"Availability and expectations of significant individuals, such as spouse, friends, and caregivers. Also includes larger social groups which are influential in establishing norms, role expectations, and social routines" (AOTA, 1994, p. 1054).

Social participation (an area of occupation)

"Organized patterns of behavior that are characteristic and expected of an individual in a given position within a social system" (Mosey, 1996, p. 340). (See Appendix, Table 1, for definitions of terms.)

• Community

• Family

• Peer, friend

Spiritual (a context)

The fundamental orientation of a person's life; that which inspires and motivates that individual.

T

Temporal (a context)

"Location of occupational performance in time" (Neistadt & Crepeau, 1998, p. 292).

V

Values

"A coherent set of convictions that assigns significance or standards to occupations, creating a strong disposition to perform accordingly" (Kielhofner, Borell, Burke, Helfrick, & Nygard, 1995, p. 46).

Virtual (a context)

Environment in which communication occurs by means of airways or computers and an absence of physical contact.

W

Wellness

The condition of being in good health, including the appreciation and the enjoyment of health. Wellness is more than a lack of disease symptoms; it is a state of mental and physical balance and fitness (*Taber's Cyclopedic Medical Dictionary*, 1997).

Work (an area of occupation)

Includes activities needed for engaging in remunerative employment or volunteer activities (Mosey, 1996, p. 341). (See Appendix, Table 1, for definitions of terms.)

• Employment interests and pursuits

• Employment seeking and acquisition

• Job performance

• Retirement preparation and adjustment

• Volunteer exploration

• Volunteer participation

References

American Occupational Therapy Association. (1994). Uniform terminology for occupational therapy—Third edition. *American Journal of Occupational Therapy, 48,* 1047–1054.

American Occupational Therapy Association. (1995). Clarification of the use of terms assessment and evaluation. *American Journal of Occupational Therapy, 49,* 1072–1073.

American Occupational Therapy Association. (2000). Specialized knowledge and skills for eating and feeding in occupational therapy practice. *American Journal of Occupational Therapy, 54,* 629–640.

Bergen, D. (Ed.). (1988). Play as a medium for learning and development: A handbook of theory and practice. Portsmouth, NH: Heinemann Educational Books.

Brownson, C. A., & Scaffa, M. E. (2001). Occupational therapy in the promotion of health and the prevention of disease and disability. *American Journal of Occupational Therapy, 55,* 656–660.

Christiansen, C. H. (1999). Defining lives: Occupation as identity—An essay on competence, coherence, and the creation of meaning, 1999 Eleanor Clarke Slagle lecture. *American Journal of Occupational Therapy, 53,* 547–558.

Christiansen, C. H., & Baum, C. M. (Eds.). (1997). *Occupational therapy: Enabling function and well-being.* Thorofare, NJ: Slack.

Dunn, W. (2000, Fall). Habit: What's the brain got to do with it? *Occupational Therapy Journal of Research, 20* (Suppl. 1), 6S–20S.

Dunn, W. (2000). *Best practice in occupational therapy in community service with children and families.* Thorofare, NJ: Slack.

Dunn, W., McClain, L. H., Brown, C., & Youngstrom, M. J. (1998). The ecology of human performance. In M. E. Neistadt & E. B. Crepeau (Eds.), *Willard & Spackman's occupational therapy* (9th ed., pp. 525–535). Philadelphia: Lippincott Williams & Wilkins.

Fisher, A. G. (2001). *Assessment of motor and process skills, Vol. 1.* (User manual.) Ft. Collins, CO: Three Star Press.

Fisher, A., & Kielhofner, G. (1995). Skill in occupational performance. In G. Kielhofner (Ed.), *A model of human occupation: Theory and application* (2nd ed., pp. 113–128). Philadelphia: Lippincott Williams & Wilkins.

Forsyth, K., & Kielhofner, G. (1999). Validity of the assessment of communication of interaction skills. *British Journal of Occupational Therapy, 62,* 69–74.

Forsyth, K., Salamy, M., Simon, S., & Kielhofner, G. (1997). *Assessment of communication and interaction skills.* Chicago: University of Illinois, Model of Human Occupation Clearinghouse.

Kielhofner, G. (2002). Dimensions of doing. In G. Kielhofner (Ed.), *A model of human occupation: Theory and application* (3rd ed.). Philadelphia: Lippincott Williams & Wilkins.

Kielhofner, G., Borell, L., Burke, J., Helfrick, C., & Nygard, L. (1995). Volition subsystem. In G. Kielhofner (Ed.), *A model of human occupation: Theory and application* (2nd ed., pp. 39–62). Philadelphia: Lippincott Williams & Wilkins.

Law, M., Cooper, B., Strong, S., Stewart, D., Rigby, P., & Letts, L. (1996). Person-environment-occupation model: A transactive approach to occupational performance. *Canadian Journal of Occupational Therapy, 63,* 9–23.

Law, M., Polatajko, H., Baptiste, W., & Townsend, E. (1997). Core concepts of occupational therapy. In E. Townsend (Ed.), *Enabling occupation: An occupational therapy perspective* (pp. 29–56). Ottawa, ON: Canadian Association of Occupational Therapists.

Low, J. F. (2002). Historical and social foundations for practice. In C. A. Trombly & M. V. Radomski (Eds.), *Occupational therapy for physical dysfunction* (5th ed.; pp. 17–30). Philadelphia: Lippincott Williams & Wilkins.

Maciejewski, M., Kawiecki, J., & Rockwood, T. (1997). Satisfaction. In R. L. Kane (Ed.), *Understanding health care outcomes research* (pp. 67–89). Gaithersburg, MD: Aspen.

McColl, M., Law, M. C., & Stewart, D. (1993). *Theoretical basis of occupational therapy.* Thorofare, NJ: Slack.

Mosey, A. C. (1981). *Occupational therapy: Configuration of a profession.* New York: Raven.

Mosey, A. C. (1996). *Applied scientific inquiry in the health professions: An epistemological orientation* (2nd ed.). Bethesda, MD: American Occupational Therapy Association.

Moyers, P. (1999). The guide to occupational therapy practice. *American Journal of Occupational Therapy, 53,* 247–322.

Neistadt, M. E., & Crepeau, E. B. (Eds.). (1998). *Willard & Spackman's occupational therapy* (9th ed.). Philadelphia: Lippincott Williams & Wilkins.

Parham, L. D., & Fazio, L. S. (Eds.). (1997). *Play in occupational therapy for children.* St. Louis, MO: Mosby.

Pedretti, L. W., & Early, M. B. (2001). Occupational performance and model of practice for physical dysfunction. In L. W. Pedretti & M. B. Early (Eds.), *Occupational therapy practice skills for physical dysfunction* (pp. 7–9). St. Louis, MO: Mosby.

Pierce, D. (2001). Untangling occupation and activity. *American Journal of Occupational Therapy, 55,* 138–146.

Primeau, L., & Ferguson, J. (1999). Occupational frame of reference. In P. Kramer & J. Hinojosa (Eds.), *Frames of reference for pediatric occupational therapy* (pp. 469–516). Philadelphia: Lippincott Williams & Wilkins.

Punwar, A. J., & Peloquin, S. M. (2000). *Occupational therapy principles and practice* (3rd ed.). Philadelphia: Lippincott Williams & Wilkins.

Radomski, M. V. (1995). There is more to life than putting on your pants. *American Journal of Occupational Therapy, 49,* 487–490.

Random House Webster's College Dictionary. (1995). New York: Random House.

Request for Planning Ideas for the Development of the Children's Health Outcomes Initiative, 66 Fed. Reg. 11296 (2001).

Rogers, J., & Holm, M. (1994). Assessment of self-care. In B. R. Bonder & M. B. Wagner (Eds.), *Functional performance in older adults* (pp. 181–202). Philadelphia: F. A. Davis.

Rowe, J. W., & Kahn, R. L. (1997). Successful aging. *Gerontologist, 37,* 433–440.

Schultz, S., & Schkade, J. (1997). Adaptation. In C. Christiansen & C. Baum (Eds.), *Occupational therapy: Enabling function and well-being* (p. 474). Thorofare, NJ: Slack.

Taber's Cyclopedic Medical Dictionary. (1997). Philadelphia: F. A. Davis.

Uniform Data System for Medical Rehabilitation (UDSMR). (1996). *Guide for the uniform data set for medical rehabilitation (including the FIM instrument).* Buffalo, NY: Author.

World Health Organization. (1947). Constitution of the World Health Organization. *Chronicle of the World Health Organization, 1*(1), 29–40.

World Health Organization. (2001). *International classification of functioning, disability and health (ICF)*. Geneva, Switzerland: Author.

Zhan, L. (1992). Quality of life: Conceptual and measurement issues. *Journal of Advanced Nursing, 17*, 795–800.

Bibliography

Accreditation Council for Occupational Therapy Education. (1999a). Glossary: Standards for an accredited educational program for the occupational therapist and occupational therapy assistant. *American Journal of Occupational Therapy, 53*, 590–591.

Accreditation Council for Occupational Therapy Education. (1999b). Standards for an accredited educational program for the occupational therapist. *American Journal of Occupational Therapy, 53*, 575–582.

Accreditation Council for Occupational Therapy Education. (1999c). Standards for an accredited educational program for the occupational therapy assistant. *American Journal of Occupational Therapy, 53*, 583–589.

American Occupational Therapy Association. (1995). Occupation: A position paper. *American Journal of Occupational Therapy, 49*, 1015–1018.

Baum, C. (1999, November 12–14). *At the core of our profession: Occupation-based practice* [overheads]. Presented at the AOTA Practice Conference, Reno, Nevada.

Blanche, E. I. (1999). *Play and process: The experience of play in the life of the adult.* Ann Arbor, MI: University of Michigan.

Borg, B., & Bruce, M. (1991). Assessing psychological performance factors. In C. H. Christiansen & C. M. Baum (Eds.), *Occupational therapy: Overcoming human performance deficits* (pp. 538–586). Thorofare, NJ: Slack.

Borst, M. J., & Nelson, D. L. (1993). Use of uniform terminology by occupational therapists. *American Journal of Occupational Therapy, 47*, 611–618.

Buckley, K. A., & Poole, S. E. (2000). Activity analysis. In J. Hinojosa & M. L. Blount (Eds.), *The texture of life: Purposeful activities in occupational therapy* (pp. 51–90). Bethesda, MD: American Occupational Therapy Association.

Canadian Association of Occupational Therapists. (1997). *Enabling occupation: An occupational therapy perspective.* Ottawa, ON: Author.

Christiansen, C. H. (1997). Acknowledging a spiritual dimension in occupational therapy practice. *American Journal of Occupational Therapy, 51*, 169–172.

Christiansen, C. H. (2000). The social importance of self-care intervention. In C. H. Christiansen (Ed.), *Ways of living: Self-care strategies for special needs* (2nd ed., pp. 1–11). Bethesda, MD: American Occupational Therapy Association.

Clark, F. A., Parham, D., Carlson, M. C., Frank, G., Jackson, J., Pierce, D., et al. (1991). Occupational science: Academic innovation in the service of occupational therapy's future. *American Journal of Occupational Therapy, 45*, 300–310.

Clark, F. A., Wood, W., & Larson, E. (1998). Occupational science: Occupational therapy's legacy for the 21st century. In

M. E. Neistadt & E. B. Crepeau (Eds.), *Willard & Spackman's occupational therapy* (9th ed., pp. 13–21). Philadelphia: Lippincott Williams & Wilkins.

Culler, K. H. (1993). Occupational therapy performance areas: Home and family management. In H. L. Hopkins & H. D. Smith (Eds.), *Willard & Spackman's occupational therapy* (8th ed., pp. 207–269). Philadelphia: Lippincott Williams & Wilkins.

Dunn, W., Brown, C., & McGuigan, A. (1994). The ecology of human performance: A framework for considering the effect of context. *American Journal of Occupational Therapy, 48*, 595–607.

Elenki, B. K., Hinojosa, J., Blount, M. L., & Blount, W. (2000). Perspectives. In J. Hinojosa & M. L. Blount (Eds.), *The texture of life: Purposeful activities in occupational therapy* (pp. 16–34). Bethesda, MD: American Occupational Therapy Association.

Gardner, H. (1999). *Intelligence reframed: Multiple intelligences for the 21st century.* New York: Basic Books.

Hill, J. (1993). Occupational therapy performance areas. In H. L. Hopkins & H. D. Smith (Eds.), *Willard & Spackman's occupational therapy* (8th ed., pp. 191–268). Philadelphia: Lippincott.

Hinojosa, J., & Blount, M. L. (2000). Purposeful activities within the context of occupational therapy. In J. Hinojosa & M. L. Blount (Eds.), *The texture of life: Purposeful activities in occupational therapy* (pp. 1–15). Bethesda, MD: American Occupational Therapy Association.

Holm, M. B., Rogers, J. C., & Stone, R. G. (1998). Treatment of performance contexts. In M. E. Neistadt & E. B. Crepeau (Eds.), *Willard & Spackman's occupational therapy* (9th ed., pp. 471–517). Philadelphia: Lippincott Williams & Wilkins.

Horsburgh, M. (1997). Towards an inclusive spirituality: Wholeness, interdependence and waiting. *Disability and Rehabilitation, 19*, 398–406.

Intagliata, S. (1993). Rehabilitation centers. In H. L. Hopkins & H. D. Smith (Eds.), *Willard & Spackman's occupational therapy* (8th ed., pp. 784–789). Philadelphia: Lippincott.

Kane, R. L. (1997). Approaching the outcomes question. In R. L. Kane (Ed.), *Understanding health care outcomes research* (pp. 1–15). Gaithersburg, MD: Aspen.

Kielhofner, G. (1992). *Conceptual foundations of occupational therapy.* Philadelphia: F. A. Davis.

Kielhofner, G. (1995). Habituation. In G. Kielhofner (Ed.), *A model of human occupation: Theory and application* (2nd ed., pp. 63–82). Philadelphia: Lippincott Williams & Wilkins.

Law, M. (1991). The environment: A focus for occupational therapy. *Canadian Journal of Occupational Therapy, 58*, 171–179.

Law, M. (1993). Evaluating activities of daily living: Directions for the future. *American Journal of Occupational Therapy, 47*, 233–237.

Law, M. (1998). Assessment in client-centered occupational therapy. In M. Law (Ed.), *Client-centered occupational therapy* (pp. 89–106). Thorofare, NJ: Slack.

Lifson, L. E., & Simon, R. I. (Eds.). (1998). *The mental health practitioner and the law: A comprehensive handbook.* Cambridge, MA: Harvard University Press.

Llorens, L. (1993). Activity analysis: Agreement between participants and observers on perceived factors and occupation components. *Occupational Therapy Journal of Research, 13,* 198–211.

Ludwig, F. M. (1993). Anne Cronin Mosey. In R. J. Miller & K. F. Walker (Eds.), *Perspectives on theory for the practice of occupational therapy* (pp. 41–63). Gaithersburg, MD: Aspen.

Mosey, A. C. (1981). Legitimate tools of occupational therapy. In A. Mosey (Ed.), *Occupational therapy: Configuration of a profession* (pp. 89–118). New York: Raven.

Mosey, A. C. (1986). *Psychosocial components of occupational therapy.* New York: Raven.

Nelson, D. L. (1988). Occupation: Form and performance. *American Journal of Occupational Therapy, 42,* 633–641.

Pierce, D. (1999, September). Putting occupation to work in occupational therapy curricula. *Education Special Interest Section Quarterly, 9*(3), 1–4.

Pollock, N., & McColl, M. A. (1998). Assessments in client-centered occupational therapy. In M. Law (Ed.), *Client-centered occupational therapy* (pp. 89–105). Thorofare, NJ: Slack.

Reed, K., & Sanderson, S. (1999). *Concepts of occupational therapy* (4th ed.). Philadelphia: Lippincott Williams & Wilkins.

Schell, B. B. (1998). Clinical reasoning: The basis of practice. In M. E. Neistadt & E. B. Crepeau (Eds.), *Willard & Spackman's occupational therapy* (9th ed., pp. 90–100). Philadelphia: Lippincott Williams & Wilkins.

Scherer, M. J., & Cushman, L. A. (1997). A functional approach to psychological and psychosocial factors and their assessment in rehabilitation. In S. S. Dittmar & G. E. Gresham (Eds.), *Functional assessment and outcomes measurement for the rehabilitation health professional* (pp. 57–67). Gaithersburg, MD: Aspen.

Trombly, C. (1993). The Issue Is—Anticipating the future: Assessment of occupational function. *American Journal of Occupational Therapy, 47,* 253–257.

Urbanowski, R., & Vargo, J. (1994). Spirituality, daily practice, and the occupational performance model. *Canadian Journal of Occupational Therapy, 61,* 88–94.

Watson, D. E. (1997). *Task analysis: An occupational performance approach.* Bethesda, MD: American Occupational Therapy Association.

Yerxa, E. J. (1980). Occupational therapy's role in creating a future climate of caring. *American Journal of Occupational Therapy, 34,* 529–534.

Background

Background of Uniform Terminology

The first edition of *Uniform Terminology* was titled the *Occupational Therapy Product Output Reporting System and Uniform Terminology for Reporting Occupational Therapy Services* (American Occupational Therapy Association [AOTA], 1979). It was approved by the Representative Assembly and published in 1979. It was originally developed in response to the Education for All Handicapped Children Act of 1975 (Public Law 94–142) and the Medicare-Medicaid Anti-Fraud and Abuse Amendments of 1977 (Public Law 95–142), which required the Secretary of the U.S. Department of Health and Human Services

(DHHS) to establish regulations for uniform reporting systems for all departments in hospitals, including consistent terminology upon which to base reimbursement decisions. The AOTA developed the 1979 document to meet this requirement. However, the federal government's DHHS never adopted or implemented the system because of antitrust concerns related to price fixing. Occupational therapists and occupational therapy assistants, however, began to use the terminology outlined in this system, and some state governments incorporated it into their own payment reporting systems. This original document created consistent terminology that could be used in official documents, practice, and education.

The second edition of *Uniform Terminology for Occupational Therapy* (AOTA, 1989) was approved by the Representative Assembly and published in 1989. The document was organized somewhat differently. It was not designed to replace the "Product Output Reporting System" portion of the first edition but, rather, focused on delineating and defining only the occupational performance areas and occupational performance components that are addressed in occupational therapy direct services. Indirect services and the "Product Output Reporting System" were not revised or included in the second edition. The intent was to revise the document to reflect current areas of practice and to advance uniformity of definitions in the profession.

The last revision, *Uniform Terminology for Occupational Therapy—Third Edition* (UT-III, AOTA, 1994) was adopted by the Representative Assembly in 1994 and was "expanded to reflect current practice and to incorporate contextual aspects of performance" (p. 1047). The intended purpose of the document was "to provide a generic outline of the domain of concern of occupational therapy and … to create common terminology for the profession and to capture the essence of occupational therapy succinctly for others" (p. 1047).

Each revision reflects changes in current practice and provides consistent terminology that could be used by the profession. During each of the three revisions, the purpose of the document shifted slightly. Originally a document that responded to a federal requirement to develop a uniform reporting system, the document gradually shifted to describing and outlining the domain of concern of occupational therapy.

Development of the Occupational Therapy Practice Framework: Domain and Process

In the fall of 1998, the Commission on Practice (COP) began an extensive review process to solicit input from all levels of the profession with respect to the need for another revision of UT-III. The review process is a normal activity during which each official document can be updated and revised as needed. Themes of concern expressed by reviewers included the following:

- Terms defined in the document were unclear, inaccurate, or categorized improperly.
- Terms that should have been in the document were missing.
- Too much emphasis was placed on performance components.
- The concept of occupation was not included.
- Terms were used that were unfamiliar to external audiences (i.e., performance components, performance areas).
- Consideration should be given to using terminology proposed in the revision of *International Classification of Functioning, Disability and Health* (ICF).
- The document is being used inappropriately to design curricula.
- The role of theory application in clinical reasoning is being minimized by using UT-III as a recipe for practice.

The COP recognized that the practice environment had changed significantly since the last revision and that the profession's understanding of its core constructs and service delivery process had further evolved. The recently published *Guide to Occupational Therapy Practice* (Moyers, 1999) outlined many of these contemporary shifts, and the COP carefully reviewed this document. In light of these changes and the feedback received during the review process, the COP decided that practice needs had changed and that it was time to develop a different kind of document. The *Occupational Therapy Practice Framework: Domain and Process* was developed in response to these needs and changing conditions.

Relationship of the Framework to the Rescinded UT-III and the ICF

The Framework updates, revises, and incorporates the primary elements (performance areas, performance components, performance contexts) outlined in the rescinded UT-III. In some cases, the names of these elements were updated to reflect shifts in thinking and to create more obvious links with terminology outside of the profession. Feedback from the review indicated that the use of occupational therapy terminology often made it more difficult for others to understand what occupational therapy contributes. The ICF language is also seen as important to incorporate. The following chart shows how terminology has evolved by comparing terminology used in the Framework, the rescinded UT-III, and the ICF documents.

COMPARISON OF TERMS

■ FRAMEWORK	■ RESCINDED UT-III	■ ICF
Occupations—"activities…of everyday life, named, organized, and given value and meaning by individuals and a culture. Occupation is everything people do to occupy themselves, including looking after themselves,… enjoying life…and contributing to the social and economic fabric of their communities…" (Law, Polatajko, Baptiste, & Townsend, 1997, p. 32).	Not addressed.	Not addressed.
Areas of occupation—various kinds of life activities in which people engage, including the following categories: ADL, IADL, education, work, play, leisure, and social participation.	**Performance areas** (pp. 1051–1052)— • Activities of daily living • Work and productive activities • Play or leisure activities	**Activities and participation**— • **Activities**—"execution of a task or action by an individual" (p. 10). • **Participation**—"involvement in a life situation" (p. 10). Examples of both: learning, task demands (routines), communication, mobility, self-care, domestic life, interpersonal interactions and relationships, major life areas, community, social and civic life. Activities and Participation examples from ICF overlap Areas of Occupation, Performance Skills, and Performance Patterns in the Framework.

(Continued)

COMPARISON OF TERMS

(Continued)

▦ FRAMEWORK	▦ RESCINDED UT-III	▦ ICF
Performance skills—features of what one does, not what one has, related to observable elements of action that have implicit functional purposes (adapted from Fisher & Kielhofner, 1995, p. 113). Performance skills include motor, process, and communication/interaction skills.	**Performance components**—sensorimotor components, cognitive interaction and cognitive components, as well as psychosocial skills and psychological components. These components consist of some performance skills and some client factors as presented in the Framework (pp. 1052–1054).	**Activities and participation**— • **Activities**—"execution of a task or action by an individual" (p. 10). • **Participation**—"involvement in a life situation" (p. 10). Examples of both: learning, task demands (routines), communication, mobility, self-care, domestic life, interpersonal interactions and relationships, major life areas, community, social and civic life. Activities and Participation examples from ICF overlap Areas of Occupation, Performance Skills, and Performance Patterns in the Framework.
Performance patterns—patterns of behavior related to daily life activities that are habitual or routine. Performance patterns include habits, routines, and roles.	Habits and routines not addressed. Roles listed as performance components (p. 1050).	**Activities and participation**— • **Activities**—"execution of a task or action by an individual" (p.10). • **Participation**—"involvement in a life situation" (p. 10). Examples of both: learning, task demands (routines), communication, mobility, self-care, domestic life, interpersonal interactions and relationships, major life areas, community, social and civic life. Activities and Participation examples from ICF overlap Areas of Occupation, Performance Skills, and Performance Patterns in the Framework.
Context or contexts—refers to a variety of interrelated conditions within and surrounding the client that influence performance. Context includes cultural, physical, social, personal, spiritual, temporal, and virtual contexts.	**Performance contexts** (p. 1054)— • **Temporal aspects** (chronological, developmental, life cycle, disability status) • **Environment** (physical, social, cultural)	**Contextual factors**—"represent the complete background of an individual's life and living. They include environmental factors and personal factors that may have an effect on the individual with a health condition and the individual's health and health-related states" (p. 16). • **Environmental factors**—"make up the physical, social and attitudinal environment in which people live and conduct their lives. The factors are external to individuals ..." (p. 16). • **Personal factors**—"the particular background of an individual's life and living ..." (p. 17) (e.g., gender, race, lifestyle, habits, social background, education, profession). Personal factors are not classified in ICF because they are not part of a health condition or health state, though they are recognized as having an effect on outcomes.
Activity demands—the aspects of an activity, which include the objects, space, social demands, sequencing or timing, required actions, and required underlying body functions and body structures needed to carry out the activity.	Not addressed.	Not addressed.
Client factors—those factors that reside within the client that may affect performance in areas of occupation. Client factors include the following: • **Body functions**—"the physiological functions of body systems (including psychological functions)" (WHO, 2001, p. 10). • **Body structures**—"anatomical parts of the body such as organs, limbs and their components [that support body function]" (WHO, 2001, p. 10).	**Performance components**—sensorimotor components, cognitive interaction and cognitive components, as well as psychosocial skills and psychological components. These components consist of some performance skills and some client factors as presented in the Framework (pp. 1052–1054).	• **Body functions**—"the physiological functions of body systems (including psychological functions)" (p. 10). • **Body structures**—"anatomical parts of the body such as organs, limbs and their components [that support body function]" (p. 10).

(Continued)

COMPARISON OF TERMS

(Continued)

■ FRAMEWORK	■ RESCINDED UT-III	■ ICF
Outcomes—important dimensions of health attributed to interventions, including ability to function, health perceptions, and satisfaction with care (adapted from Request for Planning Ideas, 2001).	Not addressed.	Not addressed.

Note. UT-III = *Uniform Terminology for Occupational Therapy—Third Edition* (AOTA, 1994); ICF = *International Classification of Functioning, Disability and Health* (WHO, 2001).

References

American Occupational Therapy Association. (1979). Uniform terminology for reporting occupational therapy services—First edition. *Occupational Therapy News, 35*(11), 1–8.

American Occupational Therapy Association. (1989). Uniform terminology for occupational therapy—Second edition. *American Journal of Occupational Therapy, 43,* 808–815.

American Occupational Therapy Association. (1994). Uniform terminology for occupational therapy—Third edition. *American Journal of Occupational Therapy, 48,* 1047–1054.

Education for all Handicapped Children Act. (1975). Pub. L. 94–142, 20 U.S.C. §1400 *et seq.*

Fisher, A., & Kielhofner, G. (1995). Skill in occupational performance. In G. Kielhofner (Ed.), *A model of human occupation: Theory and application* (2nd ed., pp. 113–128). Baltimore: Williams & Wilkins.

Law, M., Polatajko, H., Baptiste, W., & Townsend, E. (1997). Core concepts of occupational therapy. In E. Townsend (Ed.), *Enabling occupation: An occupational therapy perspective* (pp. 29–56). Ottawa, ON: Canadian Association of Occupational Therapists.

Medicare-Medicaid Anti-Fraud and Abuse Amendments. (1977). Pub. L. 95–142, 42 U.S.C. §1395(h).

Moyers, P. (1999). The guide to occupational therapy practice. *American Journal of Occupational Therapy, 53,* 247–322.

Request for Planning Ideas for the Development of the Children's Health Outcomes Initiative, 66 Fed. Reg. 11296 (2001).

World Health Organization. (2001). *International classification of functioning, disability and health (ICF).* Geneva, Switzerland: Author.

Authors

THE COMMISSION ON PRACTICE:

Mary Jane Youngstrom, MS, OTR, FAOTA, Chairperson (1998–2002)

Sara Jane Brayman, PhD, OTR, FAOTA, Chairperson-Elect (2001–2002)

Paige Anthony, COTA

Mary Brinson, MS, OTR/L, FAOTA

Susan Brownrigg, OTR/L

Gloria Frolek Clark, MS, OTR/L, FAOTA

Susanne Smith Roley, MS, OTR

James Sellers, OTR/L

Nancy L. Van Slyke, EdD, OTR

Stacy M. Desmarais, MS, OTR/L, ASD Liaison

Jane Oldham, MOTS, Immediate-Past ASCOTA Liaison

Mary Vining Radomski, MA, OTR, FAOTA, SIS Liaison

Sarah D. Hertfelder, MEd, MOT, OTR, FAOTA, National Office Liaison

With contributions from

Deborah Lieberman, MHSA, OTR/L, FAOTA

for

THE COMMISSION ON PRACTICE

Mary Jane Youngstrom, MS, OTR, FAOTA, Chairperson

Adopted by the Representative Assembly 2002M29

This document replaces the 1994 *Uniform Terminology for Occupational Therapy—Third Edition* and *Uniform Terminology—Third Edition: Application to Practice.*

Index

Note: Entries in **boldface** indicate figures; entries in *italic* indicate tables.

About the Authors

Camille Skubik-Peplaski, MS, OTR/L, BCP, received a bachelor's in occupational therapy from Eastern Michigan University and a master's in occupational therapy from Wayne State University. She works for Cardinal Hill Healthcare System as occupational therapy practice coordinator. She has presented extensively nationally and internationally and wrote a case study of the third edition of the model of human occupation and for the *Administration and Management Special Interest Section Quarterly.* Her areas of interest are pediatrics and leadership. She lives with her husband, two children, and two animals in Lexington, Kentucky.

Chasity Paris, MS, OTR/L, received undergraduate and graduate degrees from Eastern Kentucky University and currently works with clients with spinal cord injuries or disease at Cardinal Hill Rehabilitation Hospital. She cowrote an article for the *Administration and Management Special Interest Section Quarterly* titled "Leadership in Practice: The Experience of Implementing the *Practice Framework* in a Rehabilitation Setting" and has given presentations at the state and national levels on this topic. Her interests include camping and scrapbooking. She lives in Lexington, Kentucky, with her husband, A. J., and has a baby on the way.

Dana Rae Collins Boyle, OTR/L, received a BS in occupational therapy from Eastern Kentucky University, graduating summa cum laude and receiving the faculty award for achievement, and is currently working on a master's. She has worked in long-term care, home health, and rehabilitation. She came to Cardinal Hill Rehabilitation Hospital in 2002, where she specialized in stroke rehabilitation, but she has since shifted her practice area at Cardinal Hill to outpatient pediatrics. She is certified in deep physical agent modalities and is interested in the implications of caregiving for occupational therapists. She has presented on the *Practice Framework* at the Kentucky Occupational Therapy Association's and the American Occupational Therapy Association's annual conferences. She also has published an article in the *Administration and Management Special Interest Section Quarterly.* She lives outside of Lexington, Kentucky, with her husband and two dogs and takes great pride in being a part-time caregiver for her parents as well. Her graduation date for her master's is set for May 2006.

Amy Culpert, OTR/L, received a BS from Wayne State University. She has worked in a variety of pediatric settings, including the school system and hospitals. She has presented on the local and national level on various topics, including sensory integration and vision. She enjoys spending time with her family and lives in Lexington, Kentucky, with her husband, Sean, and son, Alec.